PRINCIPLES OF
INTENSIVE CARE FOR NURSES

PRINCIPLES OF INTENSIVE CARE FOR NURSES

by Janet Missen BM BCh FFA RCS

WILLIAM HEINEMANN MEDICAL BOOKS LTD.
LONDON

First Published 1975

© Janet Missen 1975

ISBN 0 433 22080 5

Text set in 10/11 pt. IBM Press Roman, printed by photolithography, and bound in Great Britain at The Pitman Press, Bath

Contents

		Page
	Preface	vii
	Introduction	ix
1.	Nursing in an Intensive Unit – Miss R. Miell	1
2.	The Care of a Patient on a Mechanical Ventilator	5
3.	Endotracheal Tubes	28
4.	The Measurement of Arterial Blood Pressure	39
5.	The Measurement of Venous Pressure	48
6.	Some Drugs Used in Intensive Care	62
7.	Intravenous Feeding – Dr. J. T. Mulvein	90
8.	Principles Underlying Oxygen and Carbon Dioxide Transport in the Blood	95
9.	The Regulation of Hydrogen Ion Concentration and Acid-Base Balance	107
10.	Physical Chemistry, Osmotic Pressure and Osmolarity	115
11.	The E.C.G.	127
12.	The Coronary Care Unit	135
13.	The Treatment of Dysrhythmias Following Myocardial Infarction	148
14.	Cardiac Dysrhythmias	156
15.	The Kidney	180
16.	Acute Respiratory Failure	196
17.	Cardiac Arrest Outside Specialised Treatment Areas	203
	Index	219

Preface

It is with considerable gratitude that I acknowledge the help and kindness of so many friends and colleagues. Dr T. Boulton, Dr L. Baker, Dr M. Clark, Dr P. Cole and Dr J. Hamer have read through various chapters and provided a great deal of helpful criticism and specialist advice. Dr J. Mulvein has written the chapter on Parenteral Feeding and supplied the basis of that on Drugs used in Intensive Care.

Miss R. Miell was the first Sister in charge of the Intensive Care Unit at St. Bartholomew's Hospital. She set the highest standards of nursing care in the unit, combined with a very real depth of feeling both for her patients and for their relatives, and it was clear that her demand for high standards and discipline in no way diminished the respect of the nurses who worked under her. I am most grateful for her encouragement over this book and for her contribution on Nursing in an Intensive Care Unit.

I have to thank Mr David Tredinnick, the Head of The Department of Medical Illustration at St. Bartholomew's for the photographs. His was hardly a fair task. It is rarely possible to arrange equipment in clinical use to suit photographic or artistic demands, but he did his best to manipulate the environment so as to maintain the very high standards and reputation of his department.

I also wish to thank the many unsuspecting nurses who had pieces of paper thrust into their hands with requests for criticism and the demand 'Does it make sense?'. Nurses are now placed in a rather special situation in Intensive Care. Not all units can arrange to have a doctor present at all times, and the nursing staff must be able to cope with the requirements of specialised nursing care, appreciate the significance of change in the clinical state and take appropriate action where necessary, admittedly within a predetermined framework but on their own initiative none-the-less. Adequate knowledge of the basic medical sciences is essential if the intensive care nurse is to understand the problems involved in the clinical care of her patients and the underlying principles of their treatment. The emphasis on physiology, chemistry and biochemistry is made with this in mind. I am most grateful to all those nurses who have given me such encouragement and who, through their questions and comments, have helped to write this book.

I am indebted to Lawrence E. Meltzer, M.D., Rose Pinneo, R.N., M.S., and J. Roderick Kitchell, M.D., the authors of Intensive Coronary Care – A Manual for Nurses published by The Charles Press, Philadelphia. Their book is well known in this country, and I found it a tremendous help in the preparation of the chapter on Cardiac Dysrhythmias. I am also grateful to Mr Peter Cull whose original drawing was the inspiration for the one demonstrating expired air ventilation.

Finally, I would like to thank Miss Stephanie Mead for her help with some of the typing, the many colleagues who have made suggestions, given their opinions and clarified points for me, and Mr Owen R. Evans, my publisher, of William Heinemann Medical Books Ltd, who has been so patient.

St. Bartholomew's Hospital   J.C.M.
January 1975

Introduction

Nurses who have not worked in an Intensive Care Unit – I.C.U. – are not always aware of the type of patients admitted to such units or of the work done there. Comments such as 'all those machines and things' or 'it isn't proper nursing' and 'all the patients are unconscious' are still overheard. It cannot be emphasised strongly enough that the patient in the I.C.U. is heavily dependent on the nursing staff looking after him, dependent not only for his comfort and well-being, but for his life, in many cases.

Nearly all patients are frightened when they become ill. The combination of illness, a strange environment, loss of dignity, and separation from family and friends can be overwhelming, and the fear of death under these circumstances is enhanced. The burden of care therefore falls very heavily on the I.C.U. nurse. Nearly all her patients are very ill when they are admitted, and the mortality rate is inevitably high. In some cases, the patient may be so demoralised that he is unable to co-operate. Demands on her ability both as a person and a nurse are constant. Inevitably and properly, she becomes more emotionally involved and this is a fact which must be recognised and accepted. The qualities of constant awareness, patience and optimism, together with self-discipline and maturity, are necessary ingredients for the I.C.U. nurse. Fortunately for those patients who have cause to be thankful for Intensive Care facilities, these virtues are not uncommon. Once initial worries about 'machines and things' are overcome, most nurses find tremendous fulfilment in the I.C.U. whether they spend only a short period there or make it a career.

It is important to remember that some patients *are* unconscious but others may only be sedated, and it is not always obvious when they may be aware of their surroundings. In order to prevent unnecessary fear or distress, you must always assume that the patient is able to hear what you are saying. Never approach a patient without warning, or without letting him know what you are about to do. You will then avoid falling into the trap of discussing the patient in his hearing either at the bedside or at the desk, or of treating him without sympathy and understanding.

The difficulties of conversing with an apparently unconscious or helpless patient are well known. They are just as relevant with the patient who is perfectly conscious and rational but who cannot speak because of the presence of an endotracheal or tracheostomy tube. Under such circumstances, patients often become frustrated and angry; sometimes they may become depressed and their progress is diminished as a result. It is very important to avoid treating patients as if they were children, either in speaking to them or in response to their efforts at conversation or occupation. On the whole, patients should be addressed formally, as this helps to maintain communication and treatment on an adult level — but there are, of course, exceptions to this rule.

The I.C.U. is frequently a busy ward. It is very easy for it to become a noisy and uncomfortable one. Constant attendance and observation means that, without sedation, the sick patient frequently has little opportunity to sleep. Carelessness — banging doors or knocking against beds for example — and unnecessary activity or noise will diminish such opportunities that do exist.

Infection

The prevention of infection and its transfer to other patients is extremely important. The presence of ill patients whose resistance to infection is reduced, and the use of equipment and treatment which provides a potential route of infection, means that great care is necessary to prevent this. Most of the equipment used in the I.C.U. is now disposable and nearly everything is sterile, so that the possibility of introducing infection has been reduced from this aspect. Meticulous attention to details such as hand-washing (after treating one patient before moving to another, emptying urine bags etc), maintaining sterile precautions when dealing with dressings and equipment, and the careful use of no-touch techniques when indicated is the foundation of a successful I.C.U. Antibiotics cannot be relied upon to cover up for shortcomings in nursing techniques.

Drug administration

Intensive therapy usually involves the administration of a large number of drugs. Many of these are given intravenously, both to produce or maintain an adequate blood level as well as for the comfort of the patient. However, intravenous administration carries with it the extra responsibility of giving the correct dose as well as the possibility of introducing infection. The practice of repeated injection through the rubber portion of a giving-set is not recommended. The rubber is likely to be anything but clean, and multiple re-sealed puncture holes are a potential source of infection which cannot be removed by a quick swipe with spirit.

Many drugs are given as a bolus dose through a two-way stopcock inserted between the giving-set and the intravenous cannula. (Bolus — a large pill; the word is derived from the Greek bolos, meaning a clod or lump). Some drugs such as analgesics may be given in divided or incremental doses if the effective quantity or the patients' response is uncertain. A few drugs are given in an infusion — *heparin, isoprenaline* and *potassium chloride* for example are diluted in 500 ml of infusion fluid, either because they are required as a constant infusion or because the bolus method is pharmacologically unsuitable or may produce deleterious side effects. *Lignocaine* may be given as a bolus or as an infusion. Large doses (5—10 mega units) of *benzyl penicillin* used in the treatment of endocarditis must be diluted in 250 ml of 5% dextrose to avoid unwanted side effects. *Digoxin* is more effective given intravenously than intramuscularly; previously given as a bolus, it is now given diluted in 100—120 ml of 5% dextrose and run in over 20 minutes or so. This is because the bolus dose creates a high blood level for a short time, during which a proportion of the drug is excreted by the kidney before it can produce its effect on the myocardium. A lower blood level produces a smaller concentration gradient and therefore a slower rate of excretion, so that the drug has a chance to act effectively.

Whatever the mode of administration, the possibility of adding infection when giving drugs intravenously should be kept at the back of the mind. Unused portals of stopcocks should be sealed, e.g. with sterile bungs such as the Braunule; hands should be washed before drawing up drugs and injecting them through stopcocks or into infusion bottles; the caps of infusion bottles should be sprayed with spirit before puncture; and the aim at all times should be to maintain a 'no-touch' technique—keeping the fingers well away from the caps of infusion bottles, the edges of broken-open ampules and, in particular, the shafts of giving-set needles. Ideally, infusion bottles should be sprayed with spirit before puncture; and the aim at all infusion from any one bottle should be completed by the end of 8 hours. If drugs have to be added to the bottle, infection is more likely when this is done on the ward rather than under sterile conditions in the pharmacy. In the case of potassium chloride, bottles of both normal saline and 5% dextrose containing 20, 40, and 60 mEq (milliequivalents) are now commercially available. Dilutions of heparin however have a short life so cannot be prepared in advance, and although lignocaine is frequently used as a dilution of 500 mg in 500 ml for the treatment of ventricular ectopics, it is often required in other dilutions for this condition and prepared solutions are not a practical proposition.

Administration

This varies from one unit to another. In some, a specialist in Intensive Care is in charge, and is responsible for the patients while they are in the unit as well as for their admission and discharge. In other units, patients remain under the supervision of the member of the consultant staff under whose care they were first admitted, but the administration of the unit, and any necessary arbitration over admissions, is vested in one consultant only.

Not all units are able to retain a junior member of the medical staff to be based on the unit and be responsible for the daily management of the patients there. In some ways this is the ideal situation. One person provides continuity, which is important — and helpful to the nursing staff — particularly when the patient is likely to be seen by a number of specialists. Being free from all other commitments, he is instantly available to cope with any emergencies when they occur, and confusion is less likely if all instructions or changes in treatment are channelled through one person. If this is not possible, it is important that:

1) routine visits by junior medical staff are made early in the morning so that specimens for the laboratory or requests for investigations may be collected and despatched in good time.
2) the patient's notes are comprehensive and kept up to date. Housemen have many duties and are not always available to present a case to a visiting consultant, and it is not fair to expect the nursing staff to do this.
3) instructions are clearly written down
4) any such instructions are brought to the notice of the Sister in charge before the author leaves the unit.

Liaison with other departments

Pathological specimens are likely to be required and despatched to the laboratory at any time, apart from those required routinely. They may be collected by the nursing staff, pathology or other technicians, or the medical staff, but in most cases, it will be the nursing staff who make the necessary arrangements. Good quality portable X-rays are also liable to be needed at short notice, apart from daily chest X-rays which are necessary for patients on mechanical ventilators in the initial stages of treatment. Extra visits from the unit physiotherapist may also be required. An efficient and mutually sympathetic liaison between the I.C.U. and these very busy departments is important and involves both nursing and medical staff. A moment spent explaining the background to a request 'out of hours' for example is never wasted.

The pathology, X-ray and physiotherapy departments play a vital role

in the successful management of patients in the I.C.U. Their varying
functions require co-ordination however. Work on specimens for routine
laboratory investigation commonly starts at 1000 hours so that the
specimens must have arrived in the laboratory by this time. Chest X-rays
take at least 5 minutes per patient and since the radiographer must wait
until everyone is safely out of the way before exposing her film, other
procedures will be constantly interrupted until the radiographer has
finished. Collection of blood samples will be completed more quickly,
and physiotherapy will be more effective, if permitted to proceed un-
interrupted. Physiotherapy tends to tire the patient so it is preferable
to do this last of all in order that the patients can rest for a while afterwards. The Sister in charge will try to arrange early morning work to
take account of all these factors — as well as the visits of the medical
staff.

It is obvious that a considerable amount of activity takes place between
0800 and 1000 hours. One potential hazard is that routine observations
can easily be neglected or overlooked so that the patients may be at
greater risk during this period.

Charts

A large number of charts are used in the I.C.U. The type, design and size
vary from unit to unit. However clear and well-defined the chart, it
cannot always be expected to present an 'instant picture' to visiting
medical staff — and charts are more difficult to understand if they are
not filled in as neatly as possible. Charts are important, however. They
will frequently confirm a change in condition over a period of time
that may only be suspected in the first instance. Accurate assessment of
fluid balance is impossible without them, and they also play a part in
maintaining a check on routine treatment and the effects of drug administration. They are also helpful, if well kept, in providing a review of
previous progress when specialists are called in to give advice.

Duration of stay in the I.C.U.

It has become increasingly common for patients to be returned to the
I.C.U. following emergency surgery particularly during the night when
facilities and trained staff are limited. Constant observation for the first
24 hours following certain surgical procedures or on poor risk patients
can impose a heavy burden on the general wards, and some surgeons
may send certain cases to the I.C.U. on this account. Some hospitals use
a Recovery area combined with and staffed by the I.C.U. to which all
patients are returned following surgery; in some cases, the patients remain
only until they are fully conscious — in others, they may remain until the

following day when their condition may be expected to be stable and the need for the care of trained nurses is slightly reduced. This practice emphasises the difficulties of providing trained nursing staff in general wards at all times, and is regarded by some as proof of the necessity for establishing the principle of Progressive Patient Care in the hospital service.

Patients sent to the I.C.U. for immediate post-operative care are usually returned to the general wards within 24—48 hours but a few may require a longer stay. Although using the I.C.U. in this way creates quite a lot of extra work, the care of surgical patients who may be expected to make a successful recovery provides a stimulus to morale in a unit where morbidity and mortality rates are inevitably high, and for this reason should be encouraged. Apart from uncomplicated post-operative surgical cases, the average duration of stay is between one and five days in most units. Discharges from the unit is ideally the result of mutual consent between the staff of the unit and the general ward. A bed occupancy of 60% is regarded as acceptable for an I.C.U. because of the unavoidable fluctuations in demand for its services — in many cases however, a higher bed occupancy can be achieved.

Continuity of Care

One of the most bitter critiscisms of the concept of Intensive Care has been that a nurse no longer has complete continuity of care for her patient. Up to a point this is true. However, medical treatment has changed dramatically over the last 20 years and one result is the necessity for a considerable degree of scientific and technical practice on the part of both medical and nursing staff. This demand is not limited to specialist hospitals or techniques. For example, major surgery is performed on elderly or sick patients who could not have been considered for operation a few years ago, and many who would otherwise have died now recover. The nursing care necessary to support these patients requires trained nurses — and it is an inescapable fact that there is a shortage not only of nurses in general but of trained nurses in particular. It is not only the desire to provide Intensive Care facilities for those patients who really need them, but necessity which forces us to concentrate trained nurses in areas such as the I.C.U. and other specialised units. But this does not mean that the traditional concept of care for the patient must be sacrificed on the altar of scientific technology; the patient needs the nurse who cares more than ever before. Frequently, patients have no recollection of their stay in the I.C.U. During the immediate post-operative period, it is 'nurse' whose care, skill and sympathy they need rather than that of an individual. It is after this period, when he has to make efforts to help himself, that the patient needs the continuity and psychological support from familiar nursing staff; this aspect of nursing care is not denied him in spite of the shortage of nurses and the effects of the 40 hour week, although the continuity is somewhat modified, owing to the necessary rota system required. Indeed, patients can find it difficult these days to identify the nurses on the wards — it was much simpler when a nurse was either a day nurse, a night nurse or off-duty! It is not for me however to enter into a discussion of the nurses' role in the care of her patient — vocation is an unfashionable word these days — but I will venture to suggest that it *is* possible to fulfil the requirements of modern medical practice without losing that capacity for thoughtfulness, understanding and gentleness that is such a vital part of a nurses work.

1

Nursing in an Intensive Care Unit

R. Miell

Nursing in an Intensive Care Unit is stimulating, interesting and rewarding. In these days of very early mobilisation it is often the only place where total nursing care is required for any length of time. Staffing an Intensive Care Unit — almost always abbreviated to I.C.U. — is extravagant particularly if the hospital does not operate a Progressive Patient Care system. Sometimes owing to the fluctuation in work load, there are excessive numbers of staff: this gives an opportunity for more theoretical teaching than is possible when the Unit is working to its full capacity. The numbers of staff must be gauged on the assumption that the ward will be working at maximum capacity all the time. During slack periods surplus nursing staff may be lent to other departments at the discretion of the Sister in charge, but the I.C.U. must never be regarded as a pool from which nurses may be borrowed at will. The current staffing requirement of the Unit is not always obvious to administrators.

Some units do not have student nurses working as team members. I feel that Intensive Care is an essential part of their training and a minimum stay of six weeks is necessary. Student nurses will, of course, need constant close supervision but the experience and confidence they gain during this time is invaluable. It is not a good idea however to have students before their second year. Until this time they rarely have had enough experience of sick people on the wards and are very apprehensive about all procedures; even intravenous fluids and taking blood pressures can be alarming to a junior nurse, and this will make her feel inadequate and unable to be part of the team.

The number of staff required is at least 1 nurse per patient per shift. This means it is necessary to have about 4 nurses per bed as permanent staff, as well as a Sister. It is useless and hazardous to the patients to bring in inexperienced help from outside to relieve during sickness, holidays etc. so the ward should be able to cope with these situations internally. The number of Sisters will vary according to the size of the unit. One thing is obvious, however — the Sister-in-Charge must be on the spot and decisions must be taken at this level.

The length of time that nurses stay varies considerably. Student nurses need a minimum of six weeks, but because of other commitments a longer period is not practicable. The average staff nurse takes about three months to settle down and begin to feel competent and assured in her work, and therefore to enjoy it. This means that to give of her best she needs to stay longer than three months and six months or more is considered ideal.

This work can be very demanding physically and mentally. It is entirely unpredictable and the work load varies from minute to minute. It is necessary, therefore, for the staff to have a stable outlook, to be mature and capable. There is a need for utmost patience and understanding, but on the other hand firmness, tact and quick thinking are required.

Psychological Care of the Patient

Patients in Intensive Care Units are invariably alarmed and anxious. They can rarely have any preparation for their admission and are puzzled and worried by the strange surroundings and faces. This is even more so when the patient is unable to communicate or heavily sedated or unable to move. Fear, apprehension, lack of confidence and constant worry cause low morale. This may well inhibit the progress of the patient and can even contribute to his death.

It is vital that adequate constant reassurances with a simple explanation of their progress and condition is given. Patients must be kept in touch with life generally — orientated in time and place, and radio and television is a great help here. The need for repeated explanation has been found necessary — patients do not always absorb or understand the information given to them. It is the policy to treat everyone, regardless of condition, as if they are conscious and receptive to their surroundings. The nurses must be encouraged to talk to them and tell them what is happening or going to happen at all times. It is quite unforgivable for anyone to stand talking over or near a patient; what may seem to be a most harmless conversation can be completely misconstrued by the drowsy or seemingly asleep patient. The ensuing mental trauma and worry can have far reaching consequences.

If it is considered necessary for nurses to change their clothes immediately before entering the unit, then the clothing provided should resemble the general uniform. It can be terrifying to a patient to find himself in surroundings where everyone is dressed as for theatre or other such place. The general uniform gives him confidence and the nurses feel better and have a more professional attitude if they look the part.

As already mentioned, it is necessary to maintain the morale of the patient. Television, radio, talking books, even tape recorders and early mobilisation can be invaluable aids. It needs no effort to watch television, but even 5 minutes can do much to encourage the patient. One man said he started to get well after watching the Open Golf Championship. There is no doubt that the improvement in his condition was very marked from then onwards. One small child on admission smiled when she saw the television set — her first smile in six weeks, and the set was not even switched on. The 'Talking Book' from the library is also appreciated. Remarks like 'I really thought I must be going to get better when you put that book on' are not uncommon. Where possible it is also helpful to have flowers and pictures. Like the television and radio, these require no effort on the part of the patient, but do help to take their minds from their problems and thoughts. 'Apprehension, uncertainty, waiting, expectation, fear of surprise can do a patient more harm than any exertion' to quote Florence Nightingale.

Every patient must have complete privacy from time to time and beds and curtains should be arranged accordingly. At the same time, no patient should be left unobserved — but this does not mean that they have to be on full view.

Relatives

Very sick people need reassurance that their family and friends have not forgotten them, but they cannot cope with long visits or too many people. The visiting of relatives must, of course, be organised around each patient individually. However, on the whole, certain points are fairly general. It is usual for the next-of-kin to visit but visitors should be kept to a minimum, at least initially. Next-of-kin should be seen regularly by both Sister and the medical staff. To avoid unnecessary confusion and misunderstanding, it is wise for as few people as possible to discuss the patient's condition. Relatives must be kept clearly in the picture and honestly told the expected course. There is no place for platitudes or undue optimism — this is not only meaningless but cruel. Even a slight variation in wording can confuse and puzzle people.

Relatives need very careful, simple explanations before visiting. They must be prepared to see ventilators, intravenous fluids and tubes of all sorts. It is often helpful if on the first visit they simply look for a moment and then are given a cup of tea while they relax. In this way they are often able to cope much better. They do need guidance about what to do, when to visit and so on. 'What should I say? Can I speak to him? Can he hear me?' are common questions. On the whole, short visits of ten minutes or so are usually adequate at first, but no hard and fast rules can be made. For some patients, it is right for relatives to stay by them for most of the time — for others it may be better not to visit at all. In the latter circumstances although it may serve no helpful purpose to the patient to have a visitor who may be very distressed by his visit, it can be that the visitor may feel very guilty if he does not come. Understanding of their feelings will help to put their minds at rest on this point.

There should be comfortable accommodation if it is necessary to provide for overnight stays. A room which can be used for visitors to be seen by the doctor and where very distressed people can sit in quiet is essential. This should not be an office, but a comfortable sitting room where constant interruptions will not occur and which will encourage relaxation and ease of tension.

Domestic duties

We hear a lot about non-nursing duties these days, but there is a lot of cleaning in Intensive Care Units which must be the responsibility of the nursing staff. Lay staff cannot be allowed to clean ventilators and other equipment. In fact, the nurses often enjoy this work as it offers welcome relaxation as well as making complete the total care of the patient — so giving a feeling of satisfaction. It is necessary that the hospital should be able to provide adequate facilities for wall washing and general fumigation and cleaning, often at very short notice.

Medical management

There is no room in an Intensive Care Unit for confusion and indecision. It must be apparent who is in charge. Of necessity the patients are often seen by a number of doctors and it is essential that one who is based in the unit acts as co-ordinator from whom the nurses take their instructions. He should be responsible for day to day management and the ordering of investigations and treatment on the advice of the specialists. This policy ensures minimum confusion, maximum efficiency and co-operation of all concerned.

2

The Care of the Patient on a Mechanical Ventilator

Endotracheal intubation or tracheostomy is necessary to provide an unobstructed airway for mechanical ventilation but it deprives the patient of his natural ability both to warm and humidify the air he breathes. It also renders him vulnerable to infection and prevents him from coughing effectively. To minimise cross-infection, a sterile ventilator should be used for every patient and a filter placed at the air entry port.

The controls of ventilators vary according to the type and design, but all are capable of variation in tidal and minute volume and respiratory rate. The lungs are inflated intermittently by applying positive pressure to them and the method is called Intermittent Positive Pressure Ventilation – IPPV. Some ventilators are also capable of producing a sub-atmospheric or negative pressure phase in the expiratory period. More recently the ability to provide a short period of positive pressure at the *end* of expiration – a Positive End Expiratory Pressure – PEEP – has been introduced.

The patient on a ventilator cannot talk. He may also be unable to breathe at all on his own. He must therefore be kept under constant supervision both for his continuing safety as well as his comfort and well-being.

The aim of mechanical ventilation is to provide constant adequate ventilation of the lungs until the patient recovers sufficiently to be able to do this for himself. During this time, secretions must be removed by suction down the endotracheal or tracheostomy tube at regular intervals and precautions taken to avoid introducing infection during suction. Routine observations must be made to ensure that these aims are fulfilled. *Charts* for this purpose vary from unit to unit but most will include the measurement of

 Ventilation volume − either tidal or minute
 Inspiratory pressure
 Respiratory rate
 The flow rate of added oxygen if any

and indication that

 the water level in the humidifier is adequate
 the water temperature in the humidifier is correct
 any water traps have been emptied
 the patient has been turned 2 hourly
 tracheal suction has been performed at least hourly
 the patient has received physiotherapy

Unit charts usually also incorporate measurement of

 blood pressure
 pulse rate
 central venous pressure
 body temperature

and indicate any drugs administered.

The measurement of fluid balance really requires a large space if it is to be displayed clearly and is therefore best kept on a separate sheet, but this does vary from unit to unit. Further space should be available for daily management instructions, particularly where no one person is continuously in charge.

The charts used in the Intensive Care Unit at St. Bartholomew's Hospital are shown on pages 8–13 as an example.

Measurement of Ventilation Volume

The lungs and chest wall present a resistance to inflation which must be overcome by the ventilator. Air will pass into the lungs only if there is a difference in pressure between the ventilator and the alveoli. The greater the pressure difference the larger the volume of air that will flow in a given time. However, a pre-determined volume of air delivered under pressure can be considerably reduced by the presence of a leak, or through distention of the connecting tubing. A volume meter placed on the inspiratory (high pressure) side of the circuit can therefore give a false impression of ventilation volume.

The Care of the Patient on a Mechanical Ventilator

There is normally little resistance to the flow of air during expiration. A meter placed on the expiratory side of the circuit thus gives a more accurate recording of the air passing out of — and therefore into — the lungs.

Such meters are called spirometers (Latin spiro — to breathe)
anemometer (Greek anemos — wind)
or respirometers

The Wright respirometer shown in the photo is one in common use.

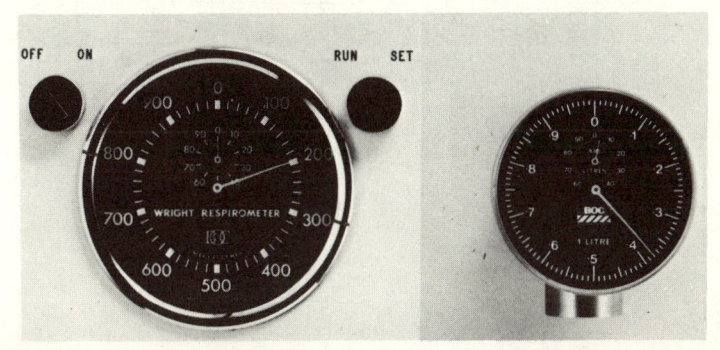

Fig. 2.1

They may be incorporated into the ventilator or may have to be inserted into the expiratory side of the circuit when measurements are made. Being made of metal, they are good conductors of heat and their temperature will be lower than that of the air exhaled by the patient. The fall in temperature (from body to room temperature) will cause water vapour in the expired air to condense and this water, if allowed to collect, will render the meter inaccurate. For this reason, the meter is left 'out of circuit' except when recordings are to be made.

The tidal volume is usually measured by recording the volume expired over ten breaths and dividing this by ten to give the average amount expired in one breath. It is more accurate to take an average than to measure a single reading. The compliance of the lungs — a measure of the ease with which the lungs can be inflated — is affected by movement, posture, coughing and straining as well as the presence of lung or heart disease. The tidal volume can therefore vary somewhat from breath to breath even if the ventilator settings remain unchanged, unless the ventilator is able to respond to or compensate for changes in compliance.

The minute volume is the volume of air breathed over one minute and equals the tidal volume multiplied by the respiratory rate. Where the respiratory rate is fixed, then provided the tidal volume remains within

INTENSIVE CARE UNIT
DAILY MANAGEMENT CHART

Date:　　　　Name:　　　　C.R. No.:

MEASUREMENTS AND INVESTIGATIONS

PATIENT	Time				BLOOD CHEMISTRY				BLOOD GASES			
Pulse					Sodium				pH			
Apical Pulse					Potassium				pCO_2			
Temperature					Chloride				St. Bic			
Respiration					Urea				Base			
Blood Pressure					Hb.				pO_2			
Venous Pressure					P.C.V.				O_2 Sat.			
Fluid Balance												
Hyperventilation												
Suction					Sputum				VENTILATOR			
Physiotherapy					Tracheostomy Wound				Tidal Volume			
					Urine				Rate			
					X-Ray–Chest				Pressure			
					X-Ray–				Oxygen			

GENERAL MANAGEMENT, DIET, etc.

TREATMENT

	Name of Drug or Preparation	Quantity	Frequency of dose	Routes
I.V. FLUIDS				
DRUGS etc.				
'A' means ADD to drip bottle				

NOTE: Drugs must also be prescribed and checked on the Blue Board. Completed by..................

DAILY FLUID BALANCE

TIME:	ORAL	TUBE:	I.V.	I.V.	VOMIT ASPIRATE:	URINE:	DRAINS:			

DAY TOTAL

12 HRLY NIGHT TOTAL
24 HRLY TOTAL

BALANCE FOR 24 HOURS:

BALANCE FOR PREVIOUS 24 HOURS:

CONSULTANT

WARD

DATE

TIME

Temperature

B.P. V
    ∧
Pulse •

200
180
160
140
120
100
80
60
40
20
0

C.V.P. cm.H₂O

TIDAL VOLUME
    V
Limits
.... ml to .... ml

Ventilating Pressure X
Prescribed Limits

Respiratory rate
(Spontaneous)

⊙

ROUTINE O₂   L/min
CHECKS   Physio
     Suction
     Hyperventilation
     Humidifier
     Traps
     Turning and Pressure Areas
     Oral and Eye Care
     Dressings

DRUGS

pre-determined limits, the minute volume must remain within a certain range also. In some ventilators however, the respiratory rate is not fixed mechanically and the minute volume, not the tidal, must be measured.

Settling a patient on a ventilator

It is usual to settle a patient on a ventilator by inhibiting spontaneous attempts to breathe. This can be done by providing deep breaths at a normal rate or less deep breaths more frequently. In either case, the aim is to over-ventilate the patient and reduce the carbon dioxide tension of the arterial blood ($PaCO_2$). Since the $PaCO_2$ is one of the factors controlling normal respiration, a reduction below the normal range (36–44 mmHg) is usually enough to prevent the patient attempting to breathe on his own. There is no need to drop the $PaCO_2$ below 28–30 mmHg – in fact a lower level can be detrimental, causing a reduced cerebral blood flow and changes in the distribution of ions, particularly potassium, which can be responsible for cardiac irregularities. Occasionally, a patient needs a greater than average minute volume to prevent him feeling that he wants to breathe. Such hyperventilation would reduce the $PaCO_2$ too far but by inserting a length of tubing between the ventilator and the patient – a dead space – the patient is forced to re-breathe some of his expired air. As the expired air contains carbon dioxide, the insertion of a dead space helps to maintain the arterial carbon dioxide level in the presence of excessive ventilation. The actual length of tubing forming the dead space volume required to maintain the $PaCO_2$ around 30 mmHg must be found by experiment, but 12″ of elephant tubing providing a volume of approximately 200 ml is usually satisfactory. See Fig. 2.2.

Since ventilation is affected by pain and anxiety as well as the age, sex and the size of the patient, a normal resting minute volume is difficult to define. Special charts or *nomograms* are available which give predicted values for tidal and minute volumes under various circumstances. In the majority of patients however, a minute volume of between 8 and 12 litres will provide adequate controlled ventilation. The results are checked after an initial period by blood gas analysis.

Remember that 1000 ml = 1 litre so that 8300 ml is the same as 8.3 litres, usually written 8.3L, and that 500–600 ml provide a reasonable breath at rest.

A tidal volume of 500 ml at a respiratory rate of 16 / minutre = Minute Volume 8L
A tidal volume of 600 ml at a respiratory rate of 16 / minutre = Minute Volume 9L
A tidal volume of 700 ml at a respiratory rate of 16 / minutre = Minute Volume 11.2L
A tidal volume of 500 ml at a respiratory rate of 20 / minutre = Minute Volume 10L

Fig 2.2

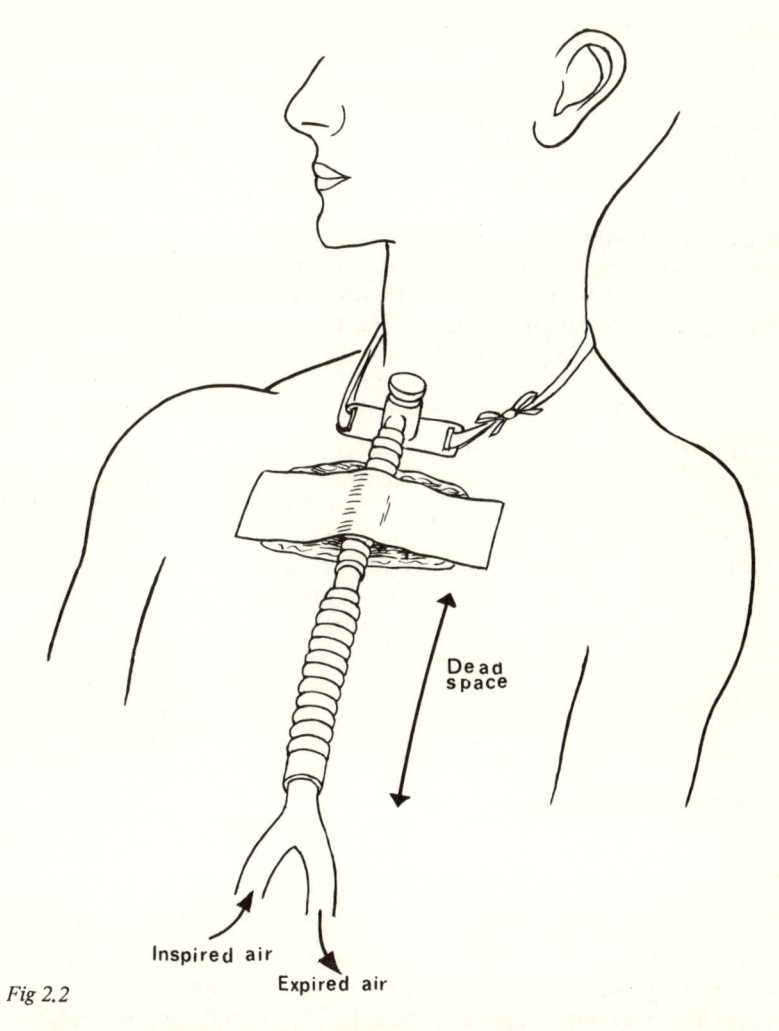

Many patients prefer to be ventilated at a faster rate with a smaller tidal volume than vice versa as this prevents them 'waiting for the next breath'. Many also prefer a regular rate i.e. a fixed rate, finding an irregular one uncomfortable and unsettling.

Some ventilators have a mechanism which allows the patient to 'trigger off' the ventilator, thus giving them a breath on demand. This has been used where the patient can make the attempt to breathe, but cannot inflate his lungs adequately in the process. If the trigger sensitivity is sufficiently responsive to the patient's efforts to breathe, it is frequently

sensitive enough to respond to the changes in pressure produced, for
example, by movement about the bed and as a result, the ventilator may
trigger off too frequently, providing breaths irregularly and often more
than necessary. If the sensitivity is reduced in order to prevent these
unwanted breaths, the patient may have to make more respiratory effort
than he needs to get a breath at all. Many units feel that mechanical
ventilation should be completely controlled until the patient is capable
of adequate spontaneous ventilation. During such controlled ventilation,
the respiratory rate should be set so that the patient is comfortable and,
under normal circumstances, makes no respiratory efforts of his own.
Provided that ventilation is adequate and the $PaCO_2$ is reduced to around
30 mmHg the average patient will allow the ventilator to control his
breathing.

Factors which will cause the patient to 'fight' the ventilator are:

1) Under-ventilation due to — the presence of secretions
   leaks in the ventilator circuit
   the development of respiratory pathology
   e.g. collapse or consolidation
2) Physical or mental stimulus — pain, discomfort, anxiety or fear
   a full bladder
   tracheal suction
   desire to cough
   emotional upset — inability to communicate, depression, anxiety etc.
3) Pathological changes — cerebral damage
   cerebral hypoxia
   metabolic upset
   low output state
   sudden onset of cardiac dysrhythmias

The presence of any of these factors must be considered and treated
whenever fighting the ventilator occurs. Often the cause is obvious and
simple and once removed, a short period of hyperventilation will settle
the patient. There is nearly always a good reason for a patient 'fighting'
the ventilator. Only if all the possible causes have been considered
and, in spite of adequate treatment, sedation or analgesia, the patient still
continues to attempt to breathe, should control by muscle relaxants be
employed. The majority of units reserve relaxants for the treatment of
uncontrolled twitching, fits, shivering or spasm leading to arrest of ventilation e.g. neurological damage, tetanus, status epilepticus and status
asthmaticus or when the cardiac output is so low or the pulmonary
pathology is so profound that oxygenation cannot be maintained even

with 100% oxygen. The patient who continues to attempt to breathe as indicated by tracheal tug, even following doses of relaxants which permit adequate ventilation, is usually in a terminal state. These persistent efforts to breathe occur in the presence of inadequate cerebral perfusion associated with poor arterial oxygenation, even when 100% oxygen is given.

The Negative Phase and Positive End-Expiratory Pressure

Most ventilators are capable of being set to produce a sub-atmospheric or negative phase during expiration. This leads to a reduction in mean intrathoracic pressure, which encourages the venous return to the heart and helps to maintain the cardiac output; however, bronchial walls which have lost their elasticity, as in chronic bronchitis, tend to collapse under the influence of a negative pressure, since this actively 'sucks' the air out of the air passages. Air is trapped in the alveoli because the bronchioles collapse before all the air can get out. In the next inflation, not only must the incoming air under pressure force the collapsed bronchioles open before it can reach the alveoli but it is then mixed with the trapped deoxygenated air in the alveoli, so that gas exchange is not efficient. Abnormal air passages together with the presence of excessive secretions make the bronchitic lung less compliant than the normal. Air flow along these narrowed passages is slower than normal (a narrow tube has a greater resistance to flow than a wide one) so that higher inflation pressures are required to ventilate the lungs adequately. It takes longer to get a breath in and out, and even restricting the negative phase to the end of expiration fails to prevent trapping. It has been shown that pulmonary and alveolar ventilation may be improved in such patients by preventing the intrapulmonary pressure returning to zero at the end of the expiratory phase (a Positive End-Expiratory Pressure — PEEP). By then most of expiration has occurred and an increase in pressure at this stage will help to keep the small air passages open ready for the next inflation. This is in fact what the chronic bronchitic does when breathing spontaneously. He breathes out through pursed lips which creates a resistance to expiration. This resistance is overcome by active contraction of the expiratory and abdominal muscles which raises the pressure inside the lungs. The forced expiration would of course lead to trapping if all the air in his lungs was to be expired, but due to the reduced flow of air, this cannot happen — he has to take the next breath whilst his lungs are still relatively full of air. By keeping his lungs more full all the time, he can reduce the amount of trapping and maintain a reasonable ventilation.

His capacity for increasing his ventilation in response to exercise is of course correspondingly reduced.

On the whole the negative phase is seldom required but it can be useful in those patients who are unable to compensate for the raised intrathoracic pressure of IPPV.

Added Oxygen

Oxygen should be added to the inspired air only in amounts necessary to maintain the oxygen tension of the arterial blood (PaO_2) between 100 and 130 mmHg. A PaO_2 consistently above normal levels is liable to destroy the lipo-proteins (surfactant) that keeps the alveoli open by maintaining the surface tension of the very thin layer of liquid lining them. Regular measurement of the arterial oxygen tension is therefore necessary in the early stages of treatment. It is desirable however to increase the amount of added oxygen before physiotherapy since ventilation stops during suction and is impeded by coughing. Care must be taken to see that the oxygen flow is returned to its former level afterwards.

Humidification

If the inspired air is not humidified, the patient's secretions whether normal or not will become tenacious and difficult to remove. Secretions tend to stick slightly to the sides of an endotracheal or tracheostomy tube; if humidification is inadequate, the stickings will dry out and act as a focus for further material. The tube will eventually block — and this can happen within a few hours. Remember too that the secretions will become sticky and viscid if the patient does not receive enough intravenous or oral fluid.

Suction down the tube only removes secretions from the trachea and occasionally the main bronchi. Coughing and physiotherapy aids the *cilial activity* which is necessary to clear the smaller bronchi, and this activity is impeded by tenacious sputum. Retained sputum not only causes obstruction but is also easily infected. The importance of humidification is obvious.

The humidifier must be checked regularly for both water content and its temperature. The majority of ventilators employ a heated water bath over which the inspired air is blown. The water temperature is maintained by a thermostat at around 50–60°C. Provided that the distance between the humidifier and the patient is not too great — say 4 ft. — the inspired air reaching the patient will have fallen from the temperature of the humidifier to the normal body temperature of approximately 37°C and be fully saturated with water, when the room temperature is around the average 24°C. The water bath temperature of 50–60°C has the additional advantage of providing constant pasteurisation and thus reduces the incidence of infection.

Thermostats can fail and allow the water in the humidifier to become too hot, even to boil. The conscious patient will usually complain about the 'hot air' but the unconscious one has no such safeguard. A simple check on the inspired air temperature (and therefore on the humidifier temperature) is to feel the metal connections between the ventilator tubing and the patient. If the metal cannot be held comfortably for at least 10 seconds, then the inspired air temperature and therefore the water bath temperature is too high. Small thermometers are available which can be inserted into the tubing close to the patient as an added safeguard.

Water traps are provided on many ventilators and some may need to be emptied regularly. They collect or 'trap' the excess water vapour condensed from the inspired and expired air. Water will also collect at the lowest point of a loop of tubing connecting the ventilator to the patient. Its presence creates a bubbling noise as the inspired air flows past it. If possible the ventilator should be arranged so that there is no loop in the tubing; if this is not possible, the loop should be drained when necessary – back into the humidifier, not into the patient.

Suction

The normal respiratory tract produces about 100 ml of sputum from the glands and goblet cells lining the trachea, bronchi and bronchioles every 24 hours. These cells and the ciliated epithelium lining the respiratory passages extend as far as the respiratory bronchioles, which terminate in the alveoli. The cells have fine hairs which rhythmically propel the mucoid sputum from the furthermost parts of the lung to the trachea, whence it is coughed up into the mouth. Normally, such a cough is appreciated only as a clearing of the throat and the sputum produced, is swallowed, but if sputum production is increased in response to irritation or infection the patient becomes conscious of its presence. Coughing involves taking a breath, closing the vocal cords and contracting the expiratory and abdominal muscles. This produces a sharp rise in intrapulmonary pressure. The glottis then opens and the air in the lungs is allowed to escape. The flow of air is so rapid that any offending foreign body or mucous is carried with it.

The patient with an endotracheal or tracheostomy tube is unable to build up such pressure although he is still able to make the attempt to cough. A tube also inhibits cilial activity in the trachea. Regular suction is therefore necessary to remove normal secretions from the trachea in order to prevent sputum retention and subsequent infection.

It is extremely important not to *introduce* infection when performing tracheal suction. Catheters must be sterile and used only once. Furthermore, disposable plastic gloves must be used to avoid infection of the hands of the *nurse*. The catheter may be held with forceps or between gloved fingers. In either case, the nurse must wash her hands afterwards. There may not be time to wash hands beforehand but provided hands are always washed afterwards, the danger of carrying infection from one patient to another will be considerably reduced. Mechanical suckers should not be shared between patients – each patient must have his own 'suction side'.

Remember that the patient who cannot breathe on his own is not being ventilated while suction is being performed. It is better to suck out the trachea quickly and allow the ventilator to provide two or three breaths before repeating suction, rather than to prolong a single effort. This is obvious where a patient's colour deteriorates within 30 seconds of stopping ventilation, but the fact of being unable to breathe for that length of time can alone cause considerable distress.

The catheter must be occluded whilst being introduced into the trachea, by bending it over the suction connection. If this is not done, the catheter tends to 'stick' to the walls of the trachea rather than passing straight down to the carina. If a Y connection is employed the open limb should *not* be shut off until the catheter has been passed as far as it will go. See Fig. 2.3.

Tracheal suction is very stimulating and the effects are similar to 'something going down the wrong way'. Some patients have difficulty in stopping coughing and they may be helped to settle more easily afterwards by being ventilated by hand rather than mechanically for a few moments. The experienced nurse, using an Ambu bag, will be able to slip in a short breath between coughs, and gradually increase the depth and rate of respiration until she has 'taken over' completely and coughing ceases. Once control of ventilation has been established the patient can be returned to the ventilator. Sensitivity to tracheal suction tends to decrease with time and the need for hand ventilation diminishes, but hyperventilation following suction also helps to reinflate any areas of lung which have collapsed owing to the negative suction pressure.

Physiotherapy

The physiotherapist plays an important role in the treatment of patients who require artificial ventilation. She usually pays at least two visits

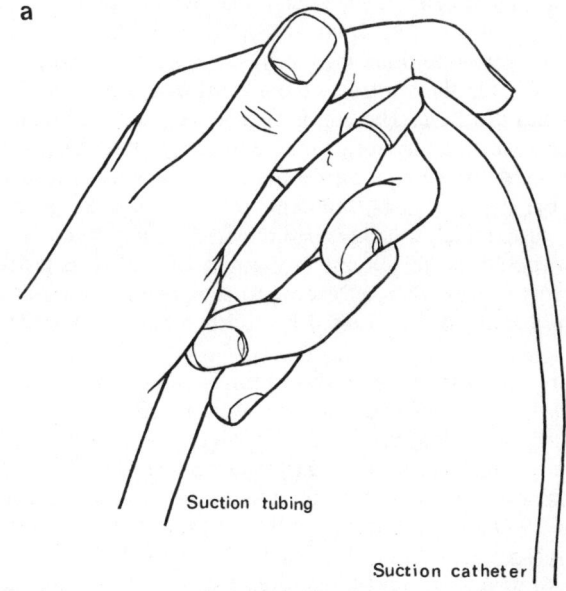

The Care of the Patient on a Mechanical Ventilator 21

Fig. 2.3a Forefinger occluding suction catheter.

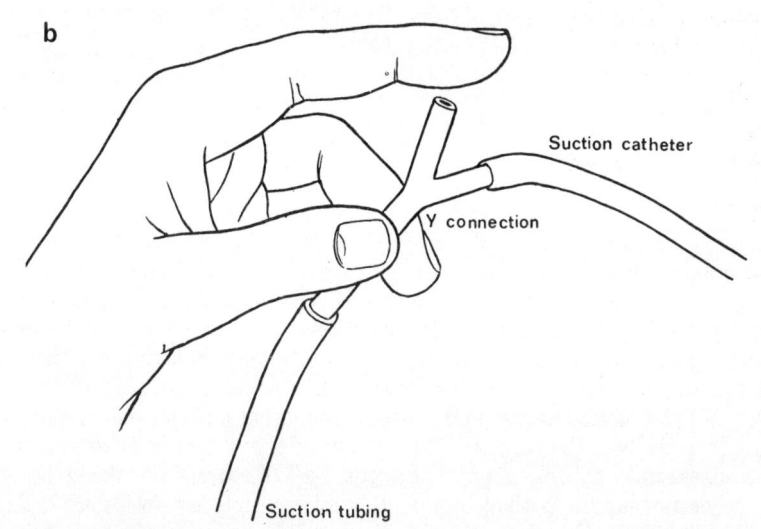

Fig. 2.3b Occlusion of the third limb of the Y connection means that all the power of the sucker can be applied to the catheter — so the third limb is not closed off until suction is wanted, i.e. when the catheter has been passed as far as it will go.

every day and more often if necessary. The patient should be placed on his side and the lungs inflated with an increased inspired oxygen concentration. This may be done manually, using an Ambu bag, or mechanically, by altering the controls of the ventilator, whichever is most convenient and effective. The aim is to achieve maximal inflation. During expiration, the physiotherapist compresses the chest, shaking it as she does so, to provide an artificial cough. She may also slap the chest with her cupped hands (tapotage) which helps to loosen any secretions — using the flat hand is painful. After half a dozen deep breaths the trachea should be sucked out in the normal way. This procedure is repeated two or three times according to the amount of secretions present. The patient is then turned on to his other side and the process repeated.

If the circulation is unstable, dysrhythmias, hypotension and arterial desaturation may occur (or be increased) during physiotherapy. The oxygen added to the inspired air should always be increased before physiotherapy commences and a wary eye kept on the ECG monitor.

The physiotherapist will also supervise passive or active movements of the limbs. When physiotherapy is finished the nurse will check that the added oxygen flow has been restored to its original setting, that the ventilation volume is within the required limits, and that the patient is settled on the ventilator and comfortable. Most patients find physiotherapy tiring and are glad to sleep afterwards. The nursing routine should be adapted to this if at all possible.

General nursing care

Position

The sick patient on a ventilator may be relatively immobile or unconscious. He must be turned regularly to prevent damage to the skin over areas of the body under pressure as well as to prevent hypostatic pneumonia and collapse in dependent parts of the lung. Change of posture from one side to the other, with a period on the back in between, should be made at least every two hours. An endotracheal tube, one or more intravenous drips, a urinary catheter and ECG leads can make turning somewhat difficult, but it must not be neglected. The conscious patient can of course signify discomfort or numbness and may only need to be encouraged to move about the bed.

Since turning the patient represents a relative upheaval in his schedule, it is both kind and good nursing to arrange that any particularly disturbing observations are carried out at this time. One of the most bitter complaints from patients about intensive care units is the difficulty of getting any sleep, particularly when frequent observation or recording is required. A little thought and quiet efficiency can help in this situation, and the continuing necessity for the timing or recording of any particular observation should be discussed with the medical staff.

It is rarely necessary to nurse the patient absolutely flat; a pillow to raise and support the head can be provided even with the most unstable circulation and if the patient is conscious, such comfort is more likely to improve his condition rather than to cause a deterioration. Similarly, as the condition of the patient improves, the 'jack knife' position can be more comfortable than simply propping the patient up on pillows, as he is less likely to slip down the bed. The raised legs will also improve the venous return to the heart if this is impaired. If a special bed is not available, the 'jack knife' position can be obtained by placing the foot of the bed on blocks and propping the patient up on pillows.

One of the virtues of this position is the fact that the weight of the patient is more evenly distributed rather than being concentrated over the ischii and the lower part of the sacrum, and this delays the onset of the 'numb bottom'.

If the patient is unable to *swallow* satisfactorily, saliva must be removed from the mouth by regular suction. The unconscious patient should be nursed on his side, the conscious patient — such as a myasthenic — may well be able to perform his own oral suction and may

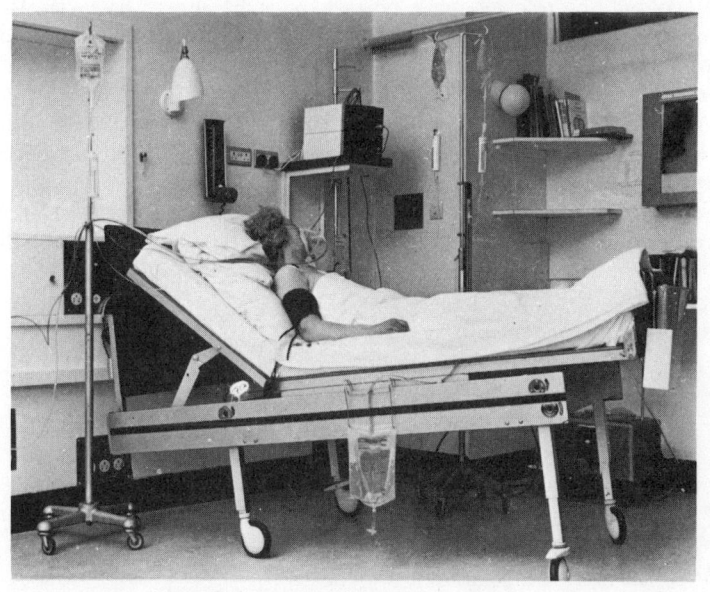

Fig. 2.4 The 'jack knife' position

therefore assume such positions as are most comfortable to him.

If the *eyes* of the unconscious patient remain persistently open, a suitable ointment may be inserted, e.g. chlorampheniol eye ointment. This has the advantage of 'sticking' the eyes shut as well as remaining effective for several hours. If drops are used, they must be instilled hourly.

Care of the *bladder*. Units vary on their attitude to catheterisation, but with closed drainage, urinary infection is not common these days and the presence of a catheter is a help in fluid balance monitoring as well as nursing care. A full bladder is also a cause of restlessness. The main danger of catheterisation is infection but the fact that most patients on a ventilator are on systemic antibiotics, at least in the initial stages, is an added safeguard. The catheter should be removed as soon as the patient can manage for himself.

Gastrointestinal tract

Intestinal activity may be reduced for various reasons; it may manifest itself as distention or require a nasogastric tube to remove gastric secretions. However, nasogastric tubes tend to stimulate swallowing, and the air swallowed can often cause discomfort. Nasogastric tubes are thus best left to drain into a bag so that air can also escape.

Nasogastric feeds must be made up with great care. Some formulae tend to be associated with diarrhoea which can sometimes be distressing and may only be resolved when normal foods are able to be taken. Hiccup occurs intermittently and may occasionally be persistent. The fact that many remedies are suggested implies that successful treatment is inconsistent.

Adequate food and fluid intake must be provided. The patient with a tracheostomy soon learns to swallow despite his tube but the presence of an oral endotracheal tube necessitates nasogastric feeding. Some units prefer to employ parenteral (intravenous) feeding right from the start if there is any doubt as to the patient's ability to take a normal diet within 24—48 hours.

Resumption of spontaneous ventilation

1) Following short-term IPPV — i.e. overnight or after 23—48 hours. The patient may be allowed a trial period of spontaneous ventilation provided that:

>   the cardiovascular system is normal — rate, rhythm, warm skin, well-filled veins, good urine output.
>   the body temperature is normal
>   pulmonary function is adequate.

Most patients can manage an hour breathing spontaneously through an endotracheal tube, although a few cannot. In such cases the tube must be removed to allow a fair trial in spite of the hazards of re-intubation if this proves necessary. A trial of an hour, or longer if the patient seems comfortable, is usually adequate to demonstrate effective ventilation, although there are a few patients who appear to be able to manage quite satisfactorily only to develop inadequacy about six hours later. For this reason, patients must be watched very carefully, without making them anxious, during this period. Humidified oxygenated air should be administered during the trial and after extubation.

Inadequate ventilation may cause obvious distress. Signs may include:

tachypnoea, (often with the use of accessory muscles of respiration), peripheral vasonconstriction, sweating, confusion or lack of co-operation, hypotension, tachycardia or dysryhthmias and diminished urine output.

Sedation is often withheld for 4–6 hours prior to a trial for fear of depressing respiration but pain and anxiety can also diminish respiratory activity, in this case already restricted somewhat by the presence of an endotracheal tube. If the patient cannot breathe effectively under the influence of reasonable sedation when this is necessary for pain, then he probably still needs mechanical ventilatory support.

2) Following prolonged IPPV via a tracheostomy.

The maxim that controlled ventilation should be maintained until all other systems are working satisfactorily still holds good. However, patients who have been on controlled ventilation for a week or more, often develop a psychological dependence upon the ventilator and may be required to be 'weaned' from it, especially if they have permanent muscular weakness as in myasthenia.

In the majority of cases, the blood gases should be within normal limits, when the patient is being ventilated with *air,* before spontaneous ventilation is attempted. Spontaneous ventilation for an hour or two — but with humidified oxygen-enriched air — should indicate whether respiratory function is adequate or not. Thereafter, the psychological aspect becomes more important. A further two hours should be allowed in the afternoon, preferably during visiting as this promotes confidence both for the patient and his visitors. Controlled ventilation should then be resumed until the next morning, when the patient should be encouraged to breathe spontaneously all day. Physiotherapy should be performed with the help of an Ambu bag. If the patient has been comfortable all day, he should be allowed to continue breathing on his own through the night without discussing the matter. If he asks to

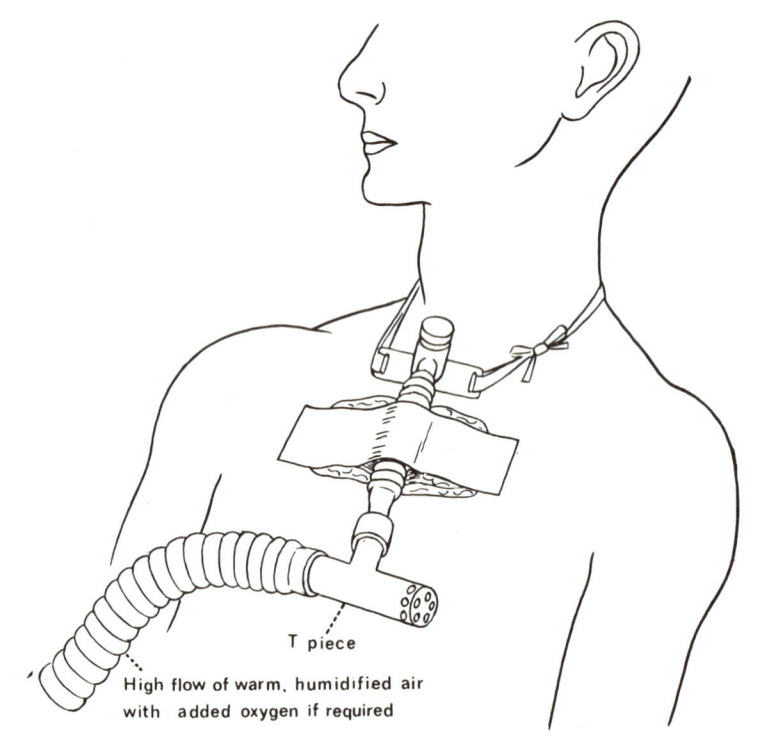

Fig. 2.5 T piece for use during spontaneous respiration. The T piece should be supported on a piece of gamgee (or the equivalent) to absorb moisture.

be returned to the ventilator however he should be allowed to do so without comment.

If the patient has breathed spontaneously all day and throughout the night, the tracheostomy tube should then be removed the next morning and the stoma covered with a dry dressing. The patient should be instructed how to obliterate the stoma with his hand both for talking and coughing. Provided that the dressing and the wound are kept clean and dry, the stoma should be closed within 3–5 days. Vaseline gauze should never be used to dress a tracheostomy; it makes the stoma soggy. Some units prefer to replace the cuffed tracheostomy tube with a small plain one, once the patient has demonstrated his ability to breathe spontaneously. The tube maintains the patency of the stoma should it be required again, and some patients find it easier to control both coughing and speech with this method.

The Care of the Patient on a Mechanical Ventilator

While the tracheostomy tube remains in place, humidified air (enriched with oxygen if necessary) must be administered and routine suction continued. Once the tube has been removed, most patients will not require added oxygen any more. In a few cases, the patient may be able to eliminate his carbon dioxide satisfactorily, but his arterial oxygen tension remains low unless oxygen is given. Such patients, usually chronic bronchitics, should be weaned from the ventilator despite the poor oxygenation as they may end up requiring permanent mechanical ventilation. Weaning in such cases may take up to 2 or 3 weeks. Patients with poor cardiac function may also take longer to resume spontaneous ventilation.

3

Endotracheal Tubes

Oral endotracheal tubes are frequently used for short-term ventilation (12–48 hours) following surgery. They *can* be left in place for 4–6 days if the patient will tolerate it and it is wished to avoid a tracheostomy if at all possible, e.g.

> a myasthenic without respiratory involvement prior to thymectomy, who might develop respiratory inadequacy during the immediate post-operative period.

> the chronic bronchitic admitted in respiratory failure as a result of an acute infection. The response to IPPV, antibiotics and physiotherapy, and the associated improvement in the cardiovascular system will permit successful extubation after 4–6 days in many cases.

When a patient is to be electively ventilated post-operatively, a cuffed *plastic* oral endotracheal tube is often used for the anaesthetic since this avoids the necessity for changing the tube later. The red rubber tubes still in general use for anaesthesia *can* be left in the trachea for 48 hours but they are irritating to the vocal cords and the tracheal mucosa. Although the response is unpredictable, the possibility of damage to the vocal cords is too great to be taken lightly. Furthermore, unlike plastic tubes which are disposable, red rubber tubes are used until they become unserviceable. Boding or autoclaving eventually makes them soft and they are then liable to kink and obstruct the airway. A red rubber tube should only be left in place:

> a) if it is felt that the hazards of changing the tube is greater than the

possibility of laryngeal trauma at the time, e.g. the cardiac arrest patient with a very unstable rhythm, requiring IPPV for a few hours only.

b) following emergency surgery if, at the end of the operation, the patient's ability to breathe satisfactorily is in doubt. A few hours IPPV will ensure adequate ventilation during recovery from anaesthesia and permit effective analgesia during this time without fear of respiratory depression. It is not unusual for a sick patient with metabolic and fluid imbalance to be unable to breathe adequately for a few hours following operation even if muscle relaxants have not been used. If however a plastic tube is readily available then the tube is better changed, under optimal conditions, even if it is expected to be employed for only a few hours.

Various points associated with the use of oral tubes:

1) Oral tubes are often difficult to fix firmly and effectively, and the method of fixation is influenced by the type of connector used. They tend to be dragged out of the mouth by the ventilator tubing and can be completely obstructed by clenched teeth unless the metal connector is so placed to prevent this happening. A sweaty or unshaven face prevents effective strapping and a firmly tied bandage tends to cut into the corners of the mouth.

2) Oral tubes are uncomfortable and provoke salivation. The majority of patients are unable to swallow with a tube in place and cannot therefore get rid of their saliva. Many try to do so which makes them gag and cough. Movement also tends to provoke this response so nursing procedures may be a trial both for the patient and the nursing staff.

Many of these problems can however be mitigated by *sedation*, which can be given freely without fear of respiratory depression because the patient is being ventilated. Restlessness, and attempts at swallowing, coughing and gagging, as well as excessive salivation, are diminished by sedation as is the liability of the tube to be displaced.

3) Suction — occasionally, and particularly with a smaller diameter tube, the passing of suction catheters may be difficult. The long tube is more vulnerable to blockage than a short tracheostomy tube so adequate humidification is essential to prevent viscous secretions. On the whole, plastic tubes are less prone to this problem than red rubber ones. They are also less liable to kink and obstruct the airway.

Oral suction to remove saliva should be performed regularly and if the tube is to be left down the trachea for more than 12 hours, a naso-gastric tube should be passed before the patient leaves the theatre or place of resuscitation to facilitate naso-gastric feeding and stomach emptying.

4) Cuff inflation — Units vary in their management. Most would agree that the cuff should be blown up just sufficiently to prevent an air leak but some prefer to allow a minimal leak. Many units prefer *not* to deflate the cuff at regular intervals because it is not possible to remove by suction saliva or debris which may have accumulated above the cuff.

Once inflated, the cuff should need no further attention. Remember that a larger tidal volume is produced by an increase in inflation pressure, so that hyperventilation used to settle the patient after suction may well produce a temporary leak. This can often be eliminated by squeezing the pilot bulb with the fingers while hyperventilating, and when normal ventilation is restored and the bulb is released, the leak is no longer present. Should an air leak occur or lead to a reduction in ventilation, the nurse should carefully add a little more air to the cuff until the leak disappears and then inform the doctor on duty as he may wish to re-assess the situation.

Nasal endotracheal tubes

Special stream-line cuffed tubes are available both in red rubber and plastic. The narrow nasal passages restrict the size of tube that can be passed, particularly if the nose is distorted as a result of a previous injury. As the resistance of a tube increases markedly with only a small decrease in diameter, it is important to pass the largest size possible. The stream-lined version can make all the difference in this respect. It is usually more difficult to pass a suction catheter down a nasal tube than an oral one, partly because the tube is longer and smaller, partly because of indentation of the tube by the turbinates, and also because of the curve imposed on the tube by the path it takes through the nose and pharynx. Nasal tubes are useful in certain circumstances such as reconstructive dental surgery — there may be considerable post-operative pharyngeal oedema in these cases which can lead to respiratory obstruction. Wiring the jaws together prevents the use of an oral tube and a nasal one is the only alternative. As ventilation is not the problem, a plain (uncuffed) and therefore larger tube can be used which will cause less resistance to spontaneous respiration.

Endotracheal Tubes

Stream lined cuffed nasal tube

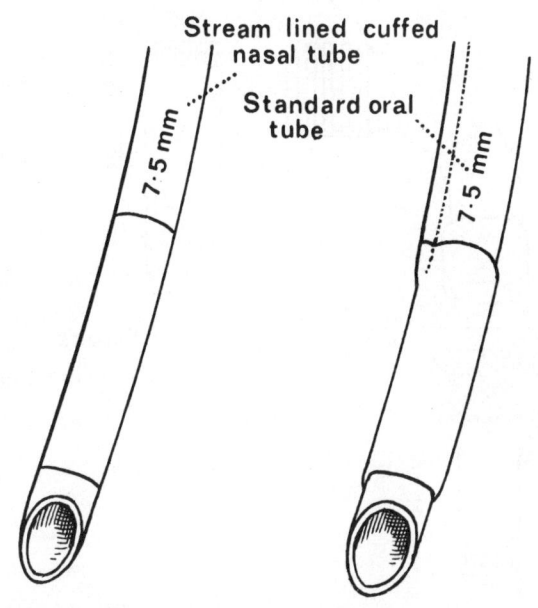

Standard oral tube

7·5 mm

7·5 mm

Fig. 3.1 The cuff inflating tube is incorporated into the wall of the streamlined endotracheal tube, whereas in the ordinary cuffed tube it lies on the outside and therefore increases the overall diameter.

Nasal intubation finds an important place in *paediatric* practice. The nasal passages of the infant and small child are larger than the diameter of the glottis and do not therefore restrict the size of tube which can be passed. The lungs of an infant or child are usually easy to inflate even in the presence of a leak, and in many cases a nasal tube is being employed to maintain a passage past oedematous tissues rather than as the means for artificial ventilation, e.g. croup. A plain tube smaller than one would use for anaesthesia will allow the child to breathe through and round the tube, or be equally satisfactory for IPPV if the need arises, and reduces the likelihood of post-intubation complications.

Methods of fixation vary from one unit to another but on the whole nasal tubes are easier to fix than oral tubes either in adults or children.

Tracheostomy tubes

These vary considerably and most units tend to have a preference both for a particular tube and its connection.

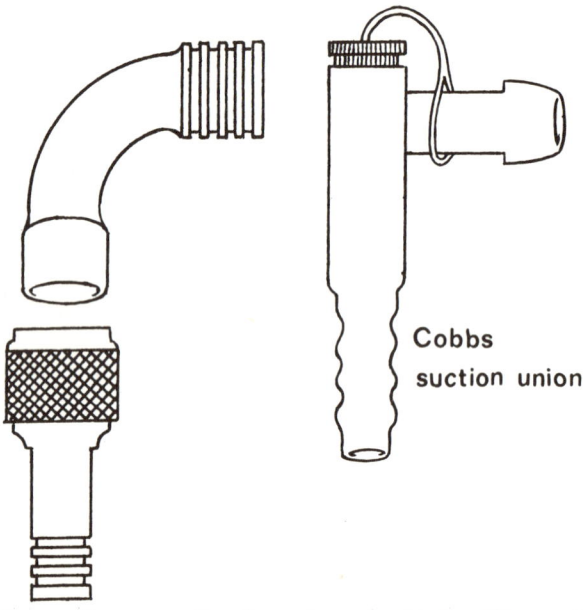

Fig. 3.2 Nosworthy connection for endotracheal tubes. The upper part only is used with the tracheostomy tube which has a Nosworthy 'chimney' incorporated.

Cuffed tubes are necessary in adults and older children if IPPV is required or if the patient is unable to swallow or cough effectively.

Plain tubes are used (1) when it is desired to keep the tracheostome open for a few days until the patient has demonstrated his ability both to breathe and swallow satisfactorily and to eliminate respiratory secretions. (2) in infants and small children. The small tidal volume involved mean that even where IPPV is required, a ventilator is still able to inflate the lungs satisfactorily in spite of the presence of a leak. A cuffed tube should *not* be used as it is unnecessary and is liable to cause tracheal stenosis.

In principle, the largest size of tube that fits snugly in the lumen of the trachea should be employed. This ensures

> minimal resistance to airflow;
> easier suction and therefore less tendency to obstruction;
> minimal cuff inflation to prevent an air leak, and therefore less tendency to produce dilation of the trachea at the site of the cuff, or eventual erosion through pressure necrosis.

It is important to prevent the tracheostomy tube 'riding forward' in the

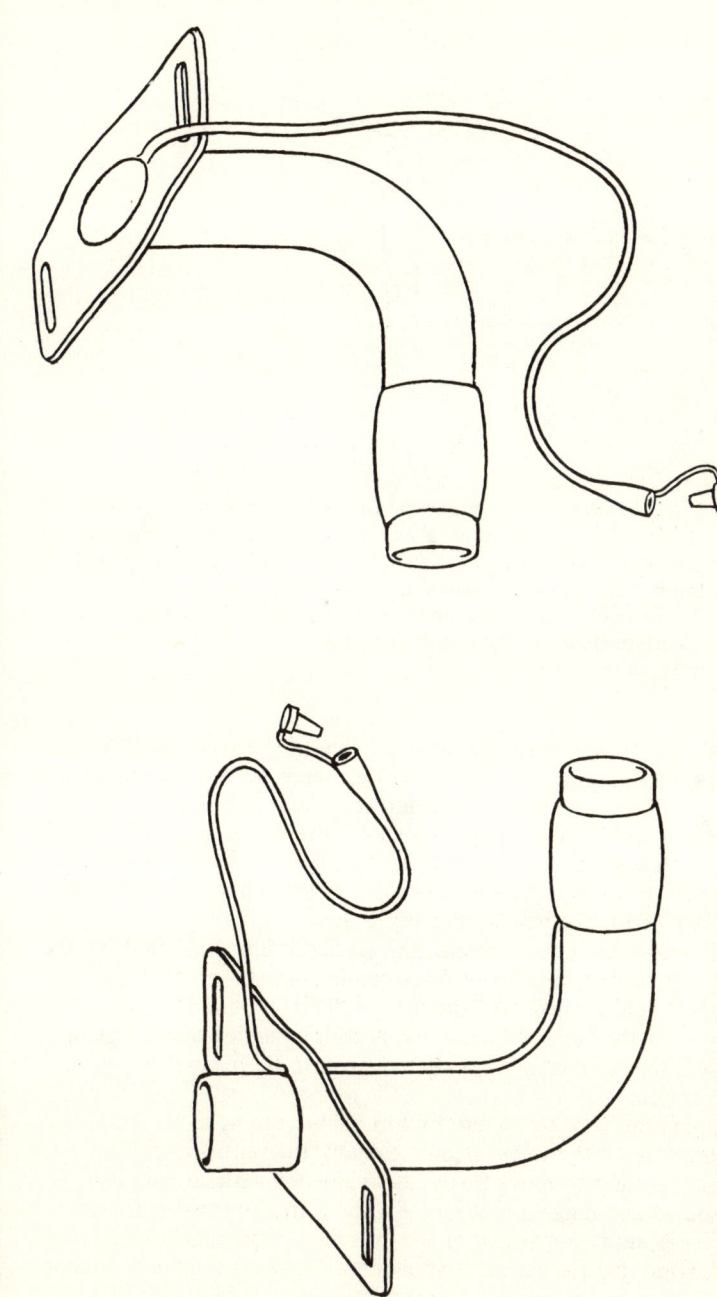

Fig. 3.2 Portex cuffed tracheostomy tubes
a) with chimney – to take Nosworthy connections.
b) without chimney, suitable for Cobbs suction connection.

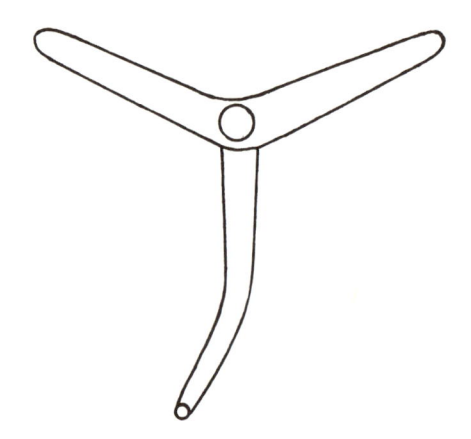

Fig. 3.2 Great Ormond Street tracheostomy tube. Infants and very young children have hardly any 'neck', so that when the tube is correctly placed, the aperture in the flange points forwards and upwards. If the wings pointed straight out to the sides, the pull of the tapes would tend to displace the tube. The backwards stoping wings facilitate fixation and at the same time help to maintain the tube in the correct position.

tracheostome. If it does so, the tube is liable to slip out under the slightest provocation and the *tip* of the tube tends to obstruct on the posterior wall of the trachea, stimulate coughing and make it difficult to pass a suction catheter. The *cuff* tends to seal off the stoma rather than the trachea so that soiling is possible and air is likely to be forced into the mediastinum causing surgical emphysema, which is both dramatic and uncomfortable for the patient. See Fig. 3.3.

To prevent these complications, the tracheostomy tube must be tied in place as firmly as possible without causing discomfort to the patient. The tapes should be tied with the neck well flexed with the chin on the chest — if they are tied when the neck is extended they immediately slacken off the moment the neck is returned to the neutral or slightly flexed position.

Strapping the catheter mount or soft rubber tubing to the chest wall eliminates drag on the tracheostomy tube by the ventilator tubing, enables the patient to move freely about the bed without pain if he is able to do so and nursing procedures to be carried out without producting unnecessary movement of the tube in the trachea. However, most units now find that the use of a swivel connection between the ventilator tubing and the tracheostomy tube makes strapping unnecessary.

Endotracheal Tubes

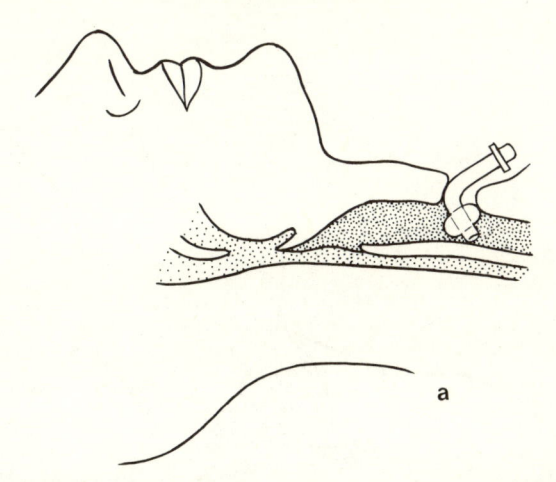

Fig. 3.3a Tube 'riding forward' in the stoma – incorrect. Note that the cuff may not seal off the trachea properly so that air can leak past and may find its way into the tissues of the neck, producing surgical emphysema.

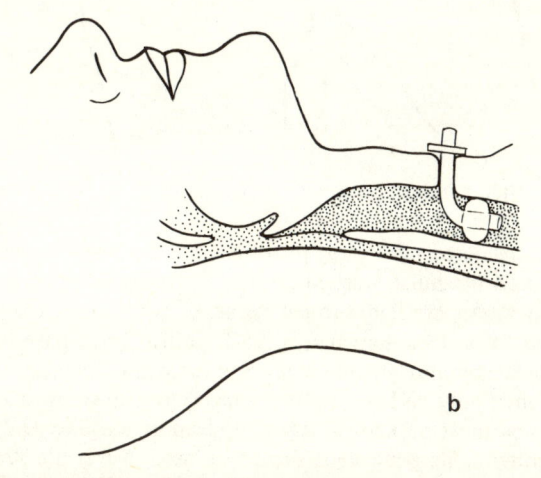

Fig. 3.3b Correct position of tube in tracheostome.

Care of the tracheostome

Infection of the stoma renders the patient vulnerable to pulmonary infection and must be avoided at all costs. Patients on IPPV should therefore receive appropriate antibiotic therapy. Tracheal suction must be performed with the use of disposable plastic gloves. Until recently, gloves

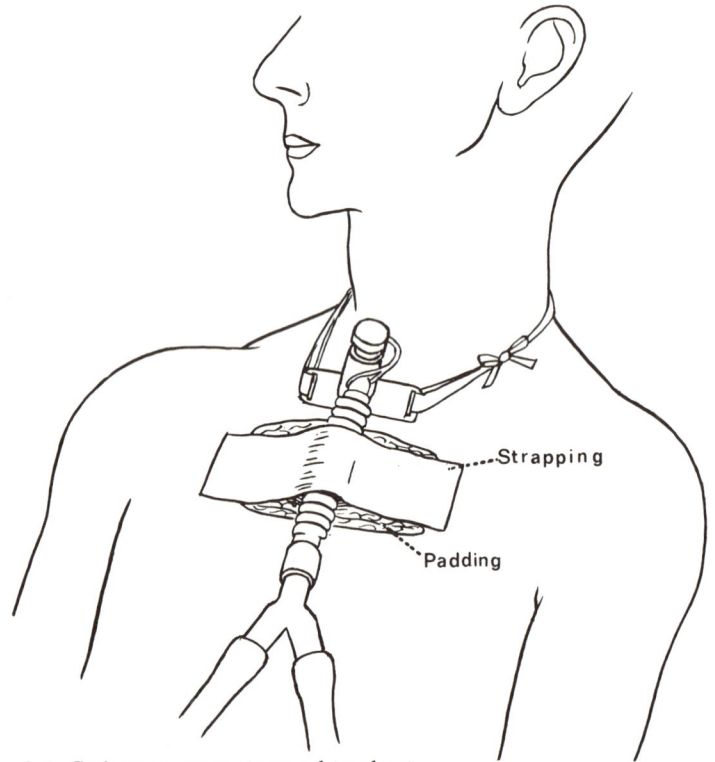

Fig. 3.4 Catheter mount strapped to chest.

were not considered necessary, provided that a no-touch technique was employed and the nurse washed her hands afterwards, but it has been shown that nurses are liable to get herpertic whitlows if they do not wear gloves to protect their hands. Each patient must have his own mechanical sucker and 'suction side'. Suction catheters must be sterile and used once only and all ancillary apparatus changed regularly.

The stoma must be kept as dry and clean as possible. Only a dry gauze dressing or its equivalent should be used. Never use vaseline gauze as this makes the stoma soggy and more liable to infection. The dressing should be changed 4 hourly or more often as necessary.

Swabs of the stoma should be taken routinely for bacterial culture — the frequency will vary from one unit to another but they are commonly taken every other day. The stoma should be cleaned first with sterile saline to remove saliva and other debris which will have tracked down from the mouth. If this is not done, the growth of normal mouth organism may obscure the presence of pathogenic bacteria.

Removal of the tube

1) *the oral or nasal tube*

Tell the patient what is going to happen and ask him to give a good cough as soon as the tube is removed. The trachea is sucked out in the normal way followed by the mouth and pharynx. With a receiver held ready for both the tube and any expectorated material, a suction catheter is then passed down the tube as far as it will go, the cuff-inflating tube is *cut* and the tube is withdrawn steadily while suction is

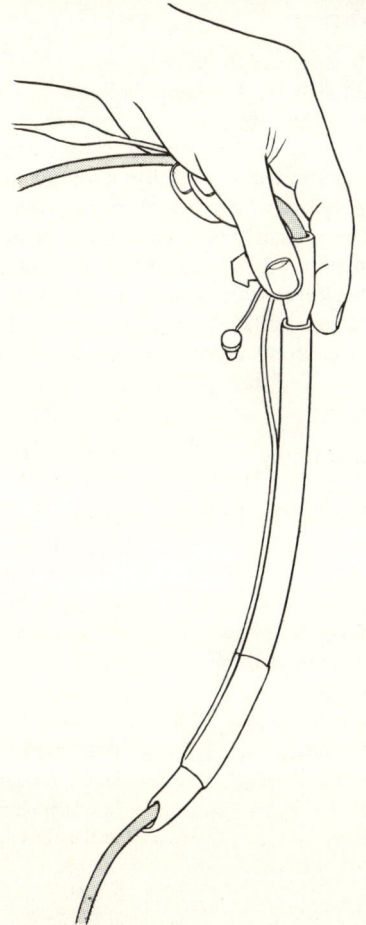

Fig. 3.5 Removal of endotracheal tube; the end of the suction catheter is allowed to 'trail behind' so as to pick up any debris which had collected above the cuff or in the hypopharynx.

applied. The tip of the suction catheter should be 'trailing' the end of the tube by about 2" so that it will pick up any residual saliva and debris in the trachea and pharynx as it passes.

The patient will almost inevitably give a good cough and produce further material. He should be encouraged to rest quietly for a few minutes, after which some deep breathing under the supervision of the physiotherapist should be performed in order to ensure maximum inflation of the lungs and the re-inflation of any collapsed areas produced by tracheal suction.

2) *the tracheostomy tube*

The patient is asked to swallow to clear his mouth and the trachea is sucked out in the normal way. A second catheter is passed, the cuff-inflating tube is cut and the tube and catheter withdrawn as before. The patient is liable to cough as the tracheostomy tube and catheter are removed, and the tip of the trailing suction catheter may be held poised at the entrance of the stoma to catch any sputum that is coughed out, to prevent it soiling the patient's skin, clothing or bedclothes. A further sterile catheter should be used for a final suck-out before placing a sterile dry dressing over the tracheostome. The patient is shown how to obstruct the dressed stoma with his finger(s) so as to facilitate coughing and speech. Provided the stoma is kept clean and dry, it should be effectively closed within 3–5 days.

Complications of tracheostomy

1) obstruction or loss of the airway	blocked tube from secretions, herniation of the cuff, malposition or kinking of the tube or catheter mount, tube falling out.
2) dilation of the trachea, which may lead to erosion	
3) tracheal stenosis	
4) erosion of the trachea	posteriorly, leading to tracheo-oesophageal fistula. laterally, resulting in massive and often fatal haemorrhage.

4

The Measurement of Arterial Blood Pressure

Blood pressure may be measured indirectly or directly. *Routine* measurement is made *indirectly* using an inflatable cuff placed round the upper arm and connected to a mercury or aneroid sphygmomanometer.

Hg – Hydrargyrum   The Latin name for mercury
Sphygmos – pulse
Manometer – pressure gauge (manos – thin, metron – a measure)
Aneroid – a not
             neros wet.

The mercury sphygmomanometer

With the valve on the bulb unscrewed, the whole system is 'open to the atmosphere' and the mercury column reads zero, since the pressure on both sides of the manometer are the same. When the valve is screwed down completely, the system becomes a closed one. If air is forced into the cuff by squeezing the self-inflating rubber bulb, the pressure within the closed system rises. Initially, the cuff will distend somewhat but the distention is limited by tail of material which is wrapped round the arm and holds the cuff in place. Once the maximum possible cuff distention has occurred, the pressure of the air in the cuff will rise and push the mercury up the think glass column of the manometer. When the pressure in the cuff is greater than that forcing blood through the arteries in the upper arm, the flow of blood ceases and the pulses distal to the cuff disappear.

Air is now allowed to leak slowly from the system by unscrewing the

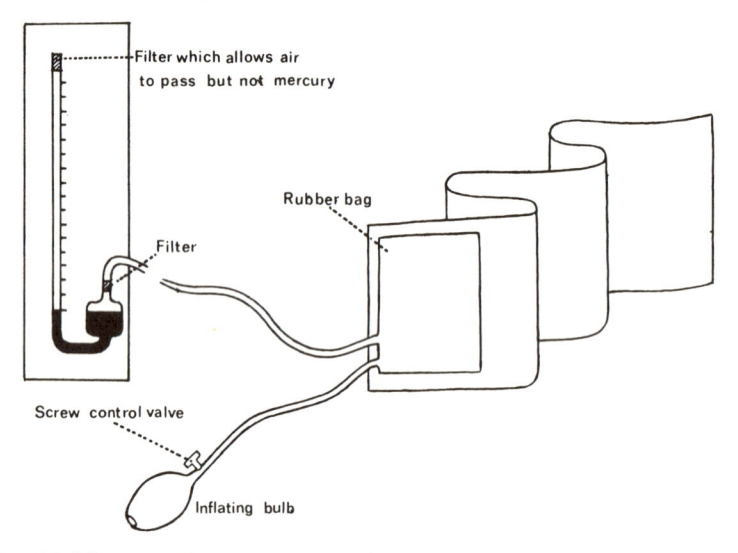

Fig. 4.1 Mercury sphygmomanometer and cuff.

valve on the bulb a little. As the air leaks out round the screw, the pressure in the system falls and the level of the mercury in the column falls with it. When the pressure falls below the arterial pressure in the upper arm, blood begins to flow again and the distal pulses reappear.

The *resumption of flow* may be determined by *palpation* of the distal pulses — brachial or radial — or by *auscultation* with a stethescope of the blood in the brachial artery in the ante-cubital fossa. The height of the mercury column, measured in mm, when the flow of blood is detected is accepted as the pressure exerted by the blood in the brachial artery, and is commonly referred to as The Blood Pressure. The auscultation method gives a slightly higher reading, as the resumption of flow is heard sooner than the fingers can detect the pulsations in the distal pulses.

The *systolic* pressure is taken as the point at which regular beats are first head or felt.

The *diastolic* pressure cannot be measured by palpation. It is taken as the point at which the regular, well-defined sounds become muffled, or as the point at which the sounds disappear altogether. The alternative is necessary because in some patients, the change from well-defined sounds to muffled ones is quite distinct whereas in others, the sounds disappear without there having been any particularly obvious change in intensity. The difference between the two methods is not more than about 5–10 mmHg.

Practical points

Always make sure that the inflatable part of the blood pressure cuff is placed over the brachial artery, on the medial or inner aspect of the upper arm. The whole cuff must be wrapped firmly and smoothly round the arm, well clear of the ante-cubital fossa. If a sleeve cannot be pushed up far enough because it is too tight or the arm is too bulky, the whole cuff will tend to slip down and become loose so that it interferes with the stethescope.

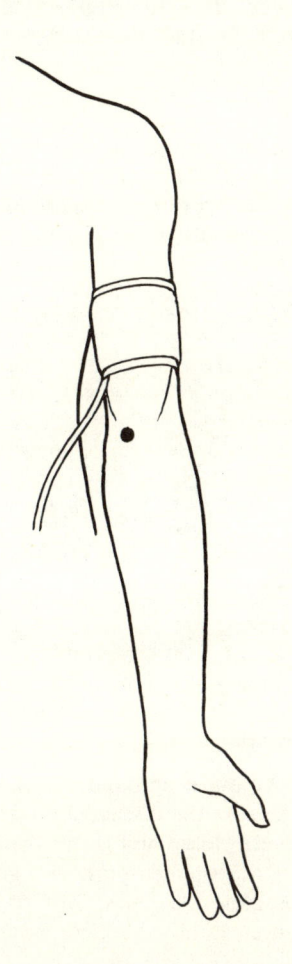

Fig. 4.2 Cuff wrapped neatly round the arm and well clear of the ante-cubital fossa.

Readings should be taken as the cuff is deflated, i.e. 'on the fall' of the mercury column. It is much easier and more accurate to detect the resumption of the flow of blood than its disappearance.

Palpating a distal pulse whilst inflating the cuff gives a guide to the systolic pressure. If the auscultation method is employed, it is wise to find the point of maximum pulsation in the ante-cubital fossa before inflating the cuff and to use this pulse to provide the guide to the systolic pressure; it can be difficult to locate the artery in the ante-cubital fossa if the patient is obese or the blood pressure low. When the pulse has disappeared, the stethescope can then replace the fingers with the reasonable certainty that the artery is underneath it.

The Oscillotonometer

Both systolic and diastolic readings can be obtained with this sphygmomanometer which employs a double cuff, one a small occluding cuff, the other a large sensing one. The occluding cuff must be above, or proximal, to the sensing cuff when placed on the arm.

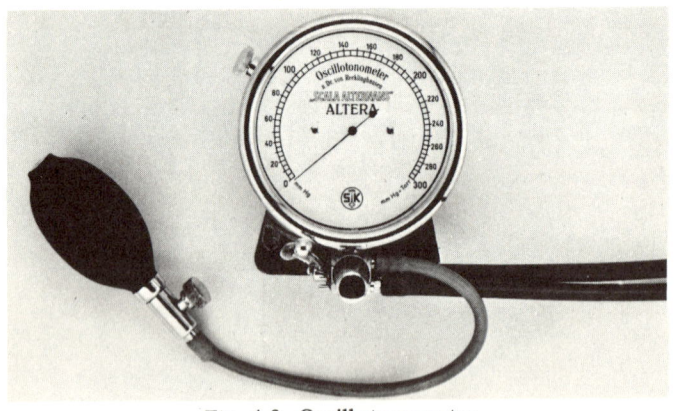

Fig. 4.3 Oscillotonometer

Taking the blood pressure

Wrap the cuff round the upper arm and connect its two tubes to the oscillotonometer. Make sure the discharge valves on the oscillotonometer and the inflating bulb are closed and then inflate the cuffs above systolic pressure, using a peripheral pulse as a guide. Then open the discharge valve on the oscillotonometer slightly to allow a small continuous leak. The blood pressure can now be recorded in one of two ways:

1) Watch the needle on the dial while the pressure drops slowly. With each heart beat, the drop in pressure is halted momentarily. As

Fig. 4.4

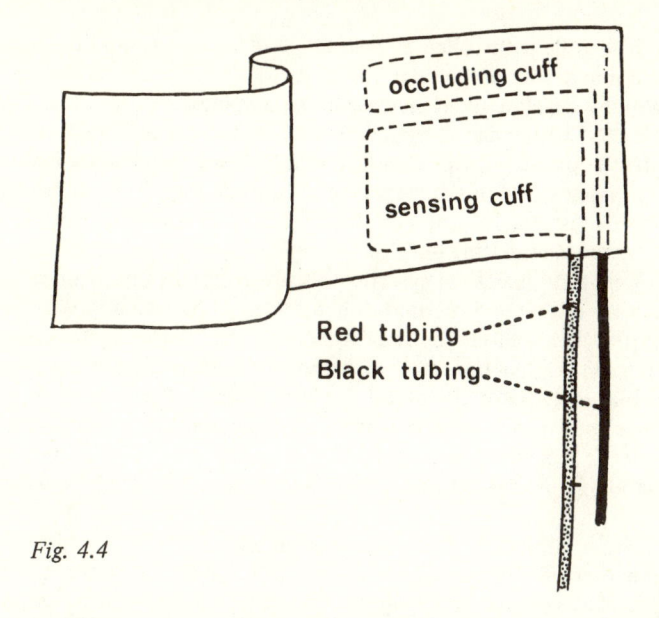

the pressure drops still further, the heart beats start to make the needle swing backwards and forwards — oscillate — as it moves round the dial. When the pressure in the cuffs falls below systolic pressure, blood starts to flow through the artery and pulsations are transmitted to the sensing cuff. At this point, the small oscillations of the needle are replaced by larger ones, and this point marks the level of the systolic blood pressure. The large oscillations continue as the pressure falls, until at diastolic pressure, they are replaced by small ones. Incidentally, the discharge valve on the oscillotonometer must be opened gradually as the pressure in the system falls, in order to maintain a uniform leak of air. When the diastolic pressure has been recorded, the valve on the inflating bulb is opened fully so that the cuff may be rapidly deflated.

Not infrequently, the change from small to large oscillations is not well marked. In this case, method 2 should be employed which makes the change more distinct.

2) Inflate the cuffs above systolic pressure and open the discharge valve on the oscillotonometer slightly as before; from now on, the valve is not opened any further, unlike the first method.

With the pressure in the cuffs dropping slowly, pull the tap handle on the instrument forwards and hold it there for a few seconds while observing the movement of the needle and the pressure it indicates on the dial.

Release the handle (controlled by a spring) and let the pressure drop a further 10 mm before pulling the handle forwards again. Systolic pressure is indicated by a well-marked increase in the amplitude of the oscillations of the needle. The tap handle is pulled forward into the sensing position every time the pressure drops about 10 mm Hg until the pressure is reached where the large oscillations are replaced by smaller ones. This point marks the diastolic pressure. The cuffs are then deflated completely with the aid of the valve on the inflating bulb.

The oscillatory change at systolic pressure is usually much more distinct using the second method, but the change in oscillations at diastolic pressure is about the same whichever method is used.

The instrument has the merit of being able to provide both systolic and diastolic readings of the blood pressure without the use of the stethescope, but in my opinion it is more vulnerable to observer variation than the auscultatory method. It does however give good results when the blood pressure is low, and palpation and auscultation become difficult.

There are a number of instruments available, based on the cuff sphygmomanometer principle, which can take the blood pressure automatically. They tend to be expensive, and false readings can be common.

Direct measurement of blood pressure

Placing a needle, cannula or catheter in an artery and connecting it to a manometer provides a direct measurement of the arterial pressure. It may be recorded simply with a mercury or aneroid manometer. More complicated apparatus, involving a transducer, amplifiers and pen writers or oscilloscopes, provides a more sensitive and accurate measurement. Whatever the method employed, a saline 'barrier' is required between the blood and the manometer.

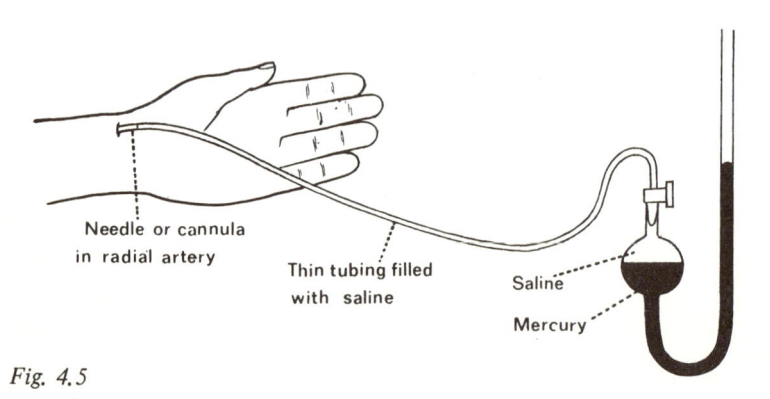

Fig. 4.5

The Measurement of Arterial Blood Pressure

The length of tubing, the saline within it and the inertia of the mercury in the manometer render the simple method insensitive. The friction and inertia of the system creates excessive 'damping' which modifies the fluctuations in pressure that occur during the cardiac cycle. Basically, the system cannot follow the fluctuations in pressure fast enough; the mercury responds to the rise in pressure during systole so slowly that the pressure has fallen again before the mercury in the column has risen very far. The mercury column falls in response to the fall in arterial pressure only to find that the pressure has risen again. The lag in response to the changes in pressure has the effect of flattening out the

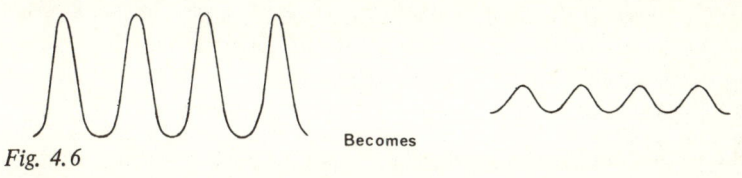

Fig. 4.6   Becomes

pressure waves and making them smaller. However, *some* damping is necessary for a satisfactory recording system; if the system is inadequately damped, it is too sensitive and even the smallest change in pressure will produce an exaggerated response.

The simple method gives only a *mean* reading of the arterial blood pressure but it can be useful when continuous evidence of arterial pressure is required. Blood will inevitably migrate back into the cannula and tubing and will clot there unless suitable measures are taken. To prevent clotting, the system must be flushed through regularly with heparinised saline. Heparin 1 ml of 1000 units per ml added to a 500 ml bottle of normal saline is an adequate dilution. Flushing may be done simply through a two-way stopcock with a 20 ml syringe. The use of a drip set allows the syringe to be re-filled from the bottle of heparinised saline and the needle to be flushed without detaching the syring from the system. The bottle of haparinised saline should be changed 6—8 hourly, since the activity of haparin diminishes with time, and in any case infusion fluids should not be administered over a period of longer than 8 hours per bottle, because of the risk of bacterial contamination following the addition of drugs to the bottle.

If a mechanical infusion pump is available, it can be used to provide automatic flushing at a rate of say 4 ml per hour.

The electromanometer

Accurate direct arterial monitoring for cardiac investigation, cardio-pulmonary bypass or intensive care problems is more reliably provided by the electromanometer. This incorporates a *transducer* which is a device for converting one form of energy into another — in this case, pressure variations into electrical variations whose energy can then be used to provide a visual or written record. Transducers are delicate instruments which do not take kindly to mishandling — being knocked or dropped, for instance. They are calibrated or set to work over a certain range and are rendered inaccurate if forces are applied to them outside this range, e.g. by attempting to flush a cannula with a syringe of heparinised saline, when the tap of the stopcock is turned the wrong way, so that the force of flushing is applied to the transducer instead of the cannula.

The advantage of the electromanometer is that, provided the distance between the arterial cannula and the transducer is kept to a practical minimum, the position of further apparatus is immaterial. The transducer must be placed at the level of the heart. Once the electrical signals have been produced, distance is no object, and the apparatus and display unit may be placed in the most convenient position, or duplicated on another screen at a central nursing station for example. They must be carefully maintained, since any leak in the system will reduce the flushing pressure and will allow blood to pass back into the cannula.

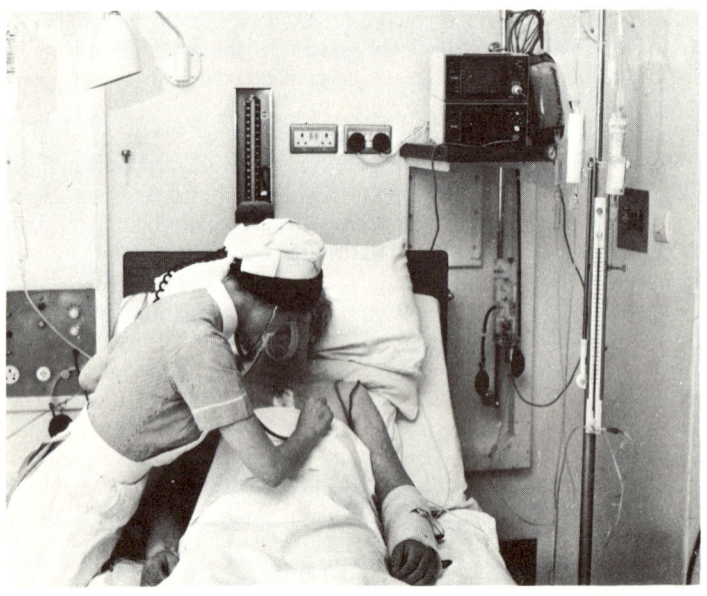

Fig. 4.7 Post-operative care showing facilities for venous pressure measurement (manometer on drip stand) and direct arterial pressure monitoring. The transducer and authomatic flushing device are incorporated in the clear plastic apparatus at the right of the headboard; the arterial pressure is displayed on the upper of the two oscilloscopes on the shelf. The lower oscilloscope is an ECG monitor. The nurse is checking the heart rate at the apex with a stethescope.

Percutaneous arterial cannulation for pressure monitoring has the advantage that the cannula facilitates sampling for blood gas analysis when required. The method is relatively trouble-free in use and should cause little discomfort or disturbance to the patient. When the cannula is removed from the artery — commonly the radial, but fine catheters are used in the brachial and other arteries as well — *firm* pressure must be applied along the artery over the puncture site, using all four fingers for *at least* 5 minutes. The site should then be inspected. If a swelling arises within 10 seconds then haemostsasis is inadequate and pressure must be maintained for a few more minutes until further inspection shows that there is no leak.

Leaks

On the whole, it is better that arterial cannulae and their connections should not be hidden under large dressings. These are not usually necessary and can absorb a surprisingly large quantity of blood before it soaks through to be observed; 200–300 ml of blood may be lost in this way. The most common cause of a leak, apart from the handle moving to the open position, is the tap becoming loose, or even parting, from its junction with the cannula. Pressure proximal to the cannula will control bleeding and permit inspection. If there is a leak around the junction, an attempt may be made to push the tap further into the cannula. This is not always successful as it is often difficult to 'get a grip' on the cannula — few have wings or any useful protuberances. If the tap has come right out, then it is probably better to remove the cannula altogether, although if the presence of the cannula is important, an attempt can be made to insert a new (sterile) tap.

Obstruction

Cannulae may become blocked in spite of regular flushing. The clot may be dislodged or the obstruction persist and require removal of the cannula. On some occasions, recording stops and although flushing appears to indicate a patent cannula, recording soon stops again. At the same time, blood cannot be withdrawn but it is still possible to inject heparinised saline. An element of arterial spasm exists here. This can sometimes be overcome by placing a hot pack on the arm proximal to the tip of the cannula and subsequently keeping the limb warm. Sometimes, gently and slowly injecting 10 mg of pethidine diluted in 1 ml of normal saline will overcome the spasm. Usually however, the spasm is the result of intimal damage and recurrence is inevitable, so that there is often no alternative to removal of the cannula.

5

The Measurement of Venous Pressure

Pressures may be recorded from both the right and left sides of the heart. Catheters, usually specially made for the purpose, are introduced into a peripheral vein and advanced towards the heart. For *right* atrial pressures, the tip of the catheter is left in the Superior vena cava (SVC) or the Right atrium (RA). To obtain *left* atrial pressures, a Swan-Ganz catheter may be used. This catheter is a flexible flow-guided balloon catheter which does not require X-ray control in order to position it correctly. The catheter is introduced via a peripheral vein into the right atrium, where the balloon is fully inflated with carbon dioxide; the catheter is then 'floated' on through the right ventricle and on into the pulmonary

Catheter with baloon inflated

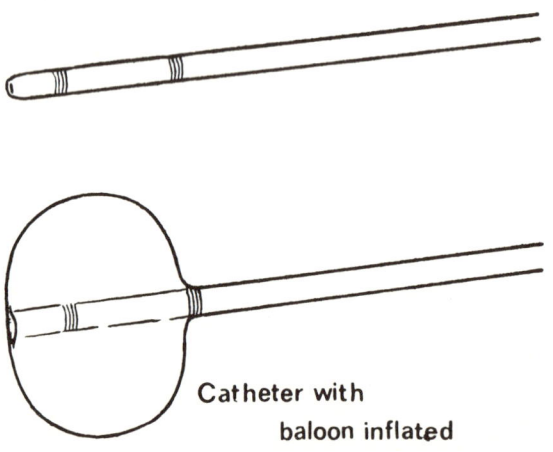

Fig. 5.1 The Swan-Ganz Balloon Catheter.

artery until it becomes wedged in a small distal branch of the pulmonary artery, thus cutting off the forward flow of blood in the artery. At this point, the catheter then measures only the pressure in front of the balloon, that is, the pressure reflected back from the left atrium. This pressure is known as a *wedge pressure*. It is virtually identical with the pressure in the left atrium and will reflect accurately any changes in left atrial pressure. The advantage of this particular catheter is that, owing to its flexibility and the balloon at its tip, it is more easily directed by the flow of blood in the heart and pulmonary arteries than the semi-rigid catheters used routinely for cardiac catheterisation. As a result, this method of obtaining a wedge pressure to monitor left atrial pressures can be employed, in the Coronary Care unit for example, without having to transfer the patient to the X-ray department.

Both techniques for measuring venous pressure are reasonably simple and the complications — infection, dysrrhythmias, thrombosis, perforation — are infrequent. The catheters can remain in place for as long as is necessary; in the case of the balloon catheter, the balloon is inflated only when readings are taken.

Where the heart is functioning normally, right atrial pressure measurement alone is perfectly satisfactory and the term 'CVP' (Central Venous Pressure) recording may be assumed to refer to this. Measurement of the CVP is often helpful where large volumes of fluid are given rapidly or where the risk of over-transfusion is a possibility, e.g. in the aged, and patients with severe anaemia or renal failure. With a normally functioning heart, it is reasonable to assume that a normal range of right atrial pressure is associated with a normal left atrial pressure. Such an assumption can be dangerous however in a patient with myocardial disease. Measurement of right atrial pressure reflects only the efficiency of the right ventricle, and it is possible for the left atrial pressure to be raised (indicating left ventricular failure) when the right atrial pressure is normal. Failure of the left ventricle is rarely immediately reflected in the right side of the heart. Only in constrictive pericarditis, where the heart is contained in a rigid covering, or in the presence of an atrial septal defect with an open communication between the two atria, will changes in the left atrium be quickly reflected in the right. The following description of the changes in the pulmonary circulation, which occur in response to a rise in left atrial pressure, is given in attempt to illustrate the dangers under certain circumstances of monitoring right atrial pressure only.

A rise in left atrial pressure results in a rise in pressure in the pulmonary veins, and, depending on the extent of the rise in left atrial pressure, will be reflected back through the rest of the pulmonary circulation. An increase in left atrial pressure great enough to raise the pressure in the pulmonary artery — normally about 25 mmHg — will impede normal emptying of the right ventricle. The ventricular volume is further augmented by right atrial contraction during diastole — so the end diastolic ventricular volume is increased, i.e. the ventricle becomes distended. If pulmonary artery pressure continues to rise in response to a progressively failing left ventricle, or to pathological changes in the walls of the pulmonary vessels causing an increased pulmonary resistance, the right ventricle becomes further distended and its filling pressure will start to rise steeply because of the stiffness of the walls of the distended ventricle. Increased force of right ventricular contraction will continue to maintain the stroke volume at this stage and right atrial pressure, although raised in order to force blood into the distended ventricle, will still only be little above the normal limit. Ultimately however, the ventricle becomes over-distended. It fails to maintain its stroke volume, and pressure in the right atrium now rises above the normal limit indicating frank right ventricular failure.

Frequently, the clinical state remains relatively static at the point where there is a moderately raised left atrial pressure associated with pulmonary venous hypertension. The right atrial pressure is normal. It is this state in which the patient is at risk when 'CVP' or right atrial pressure monitoring only is undertaken. In the normal heart, raising the right atrial pressure by transfusion will stimulate the right ventricle to contract more forcibly, thereby increasing its output, and the increased volume of blood presented to the left ventricle will produce the same effect. But if left atrial pressure is *already* raised so that there is pulmonary congestion, transfusion in an attempt to increase the cardiac output is likely to fail in its purpose and precipitate pulmonary oedema. The increased volume of blood from the right ventricle is forced into the already congested pulmonary circulation; the left side of the heart is unable to pump out the extra volume of blood, and as a result, the blood pressure in the pulmonary capillaries rises above that of the plasma proteins and forces fluid out into the alveoli.

If left atrial pressures are not monitored in patients at risk, the decision to transfuse must be considered very carefully. Routine fluid infusion therapy in patients with a myocardial infarct must also be carefully controlled in order to avoid precipitating left ventricular failure, since the presence of a CVP (right atrial pressure) line will give no indication of incipient failure of the left ventricle.

Measurement of Central Venous Pressure

Pressure in the venous system is low, so that a simple saline manometer can be used and complicated electronic apparatus is not necessarily required. A saline manometer will however only provide a *mean* value —

i.e. it is not sensitive enough to reproduce all the fluctuations in pressure that occur during the cardiac cycle. The pressure in the right atrium varies according to the position of the patient, coughing and straining, as well as changes in the circulation following infarction, haemorrhage etc. Every time readings are taken from either the right or the left side of the heart, the zero of the manometer scale must be placed at the same point in relation to the heart.

The sternal notch is commonly used as the reference point, being easily located in nearly all patients. The sternal angle may be used instead. Both are approximately 5 cms higher than the level of the right atrium and the readings are correspondingly higher.

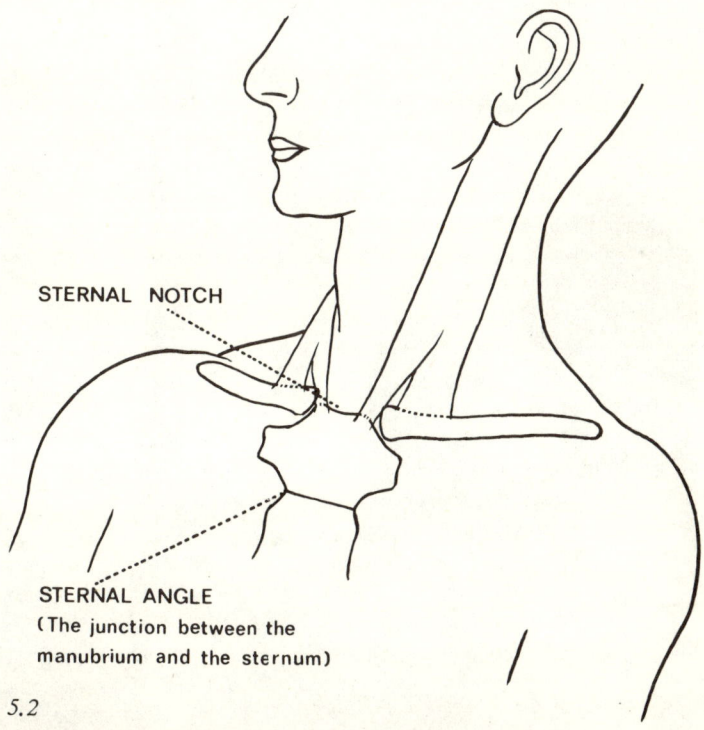

Fig. 5.2

Some units prefer to place the zero of the scale at the level of the atrium itself. Whichever point is chosen is not greatly significant. It is more important that the same reference point is used consistently to avoid confusion.

Scales and levelling devices

Paper scales are provided with the venous pressure monitoring sets made by Avon and Baxter. There are various disposable scales incorporating a manometer which may be inserted into the ordinary giving set via a three-way stopcock. A neat and light piece of apparatus is made by Becton-Dickinson (Bard Parker); this consists of the manometer scale which clamps onto a drip stand, and has a hinged extending rod at the bottom which incorporates a spirit level.

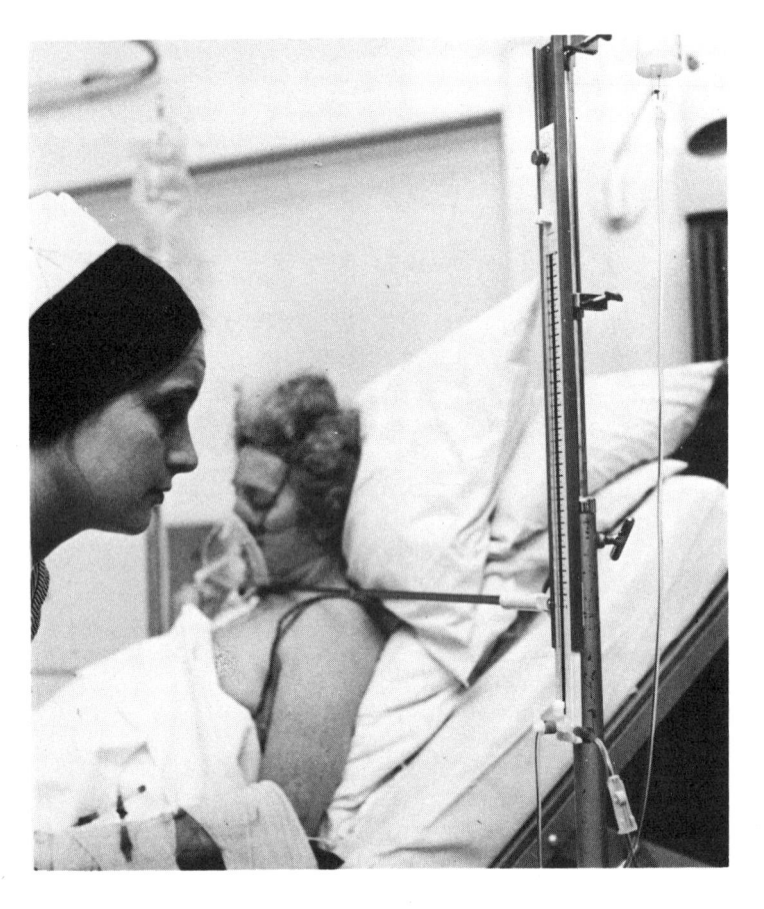

Fig. 5.3a Becton-Dickson Venous Pressure Manometer

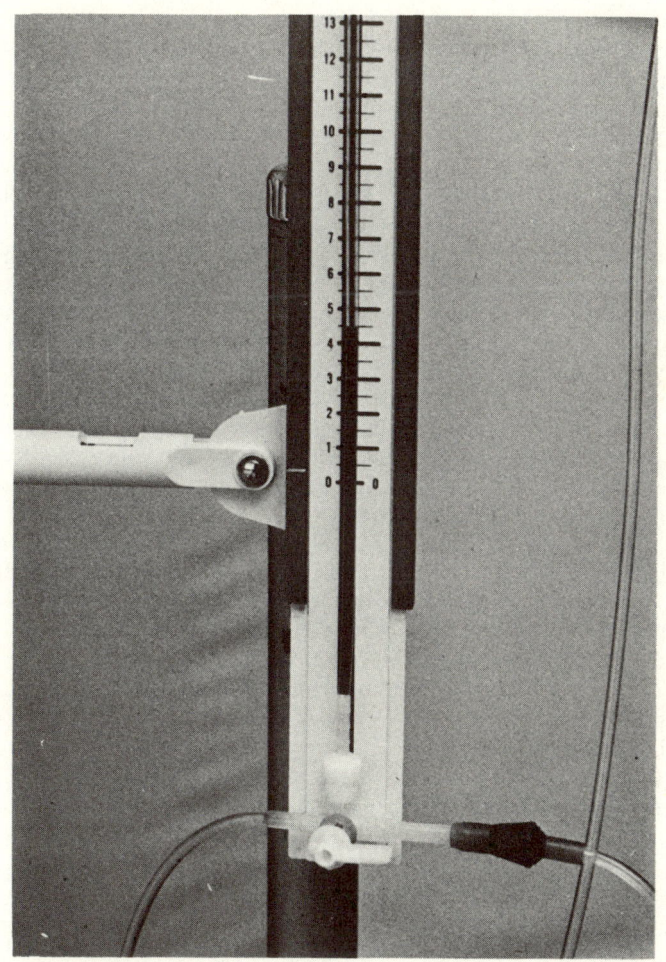

Fig. 5.3b Becton-Dickson Venous Pressure Manometer — close up.

Catheters are usually inserted percutaneously via:

the median cephalic vein	—	in the antecubital fossa
the internal jugular vein	—	in the neck
the subclavian vein	—	in the neck

Inferior vena caval catheterisation is best avoided as there is a greater incidence of thrombosis and liability of infection with this route. It is sometimes used during cardiac surgery, and the catheter left in for postoperative monitoring for 24–48 hours. External jugular veins may also be used during surgery; if a catheter can be passed on into the superior vena cava, post-operative monitoring is no problem, but frequently the catheter fails to pass beyond the level of the clavicle, and whenever the head is turned to that side, the catheter is obstructed.

A catheter at least 45–50 cms (20 inches) long is necessary for median cephalic route; 25–30 cms (10–12 inches) is adequate for subclavian or internal jugular catheterisation, and any appropriate intravenous catheter can be used for these routes. Various catheters are especially made for percutaneous venous pressure monitoring, which incorporate a radio-opaque strip. The use of any catheter threaded through a needle carries with it the risk of the needle point catching on the catheter and slicing it into two pieces, leaving the distal portion free in the vein. This is obviously undesirable and should not occur if the catheter is not drawn back through the needle at any stage during insertion. If it does, arrangements must be made to remove the distal portion as soon as possible, and may include thoracotomy. The catheters are also vulnerable if the needle cannot be detached from the system after insertion, even if a needle guard is provided. The Intramedicut (Argyl) cannula-catheter system is one which avoids this complication since the needle can be detached from the catheter after insertion. A chest X-ray is recommended after inserting a long catheter as the catheter can pass upwards into the jugular vein or even turn back on itself to travel down the axillary vein. A mis-routed catheter frequently makes it difficult to withdraw the stilette because of the sharp bends taken by the catheter. If the stilette does not come *easily,* the whole assembly should be withdrawn. Cases have been reported where the thin wire stilette has damaged a mis-routed catheter through being forcibly extracted.

The choice of route is influence by such factors as:

1) the availability and suitability of veins
2) the experience and preference of the operator
3) local custom
4) equipment available.

The median cephalic vein No special skill is required. There can be difficulty getting the catheter past the level of the shoulder. Lifting the arm out to the side, or above the head if necessary, will usually straighten out any 'kinks' in the vein and allow the catheter to be pushed on towards the heart. The Drum Cartridge Catheter (Abbott) and the Intramedicut (Argyl) are two long catheters designed especially for this approach. The catheters are soft so as to create minimal damage to the walls of the veins so a stilette is incorporated to provide sufficient rigidity during insertion. After the stilette has been removed, it may be used to estimate the position of the tip of the catheter.

The internal jugular vein is absent in about 5% people. A head down tilt is advocated in order to enlarge the diameter of the vein and to minimise the risk of air embolism.

The subclavian vein is approached from above the clavicle in the angle created by the strenomastoid with the clavicle. The needle is angled well upwards (with the patient in the supine position) which minimises accidental puncture of the subclavian artery, the pleura and the brachial plexus. The vein is anatomically constant, unlike the internal jugular vein, and successful cannulation does not require great experience. There is little risk of air embolism if the patient is lying flat.

Apparatus required

Chosen catheter
Venous pressure manometer set, or ordinary giving set, separate manometer and two-way stopcock.

Bottle of infusion fluid	Normal saline is frequently used. The drip is run slowly, being used only to maintain the patency of the catheter in most cases, so that 500 ml will usually last 6–8 hours unless the CVP must be measured very frequently. In patients with renal failure or myocardial disease, any extra sodium load should be avoided, so 5% Dextrose is used instead of normal saline.
Two-way stopcock	This is necessary if a separate manometer is used with an ordinary giving set. It is also useful if the CVP line is to be used for parenteral feeding as well as CVP monitoring, and also facilitates the administration of drugs intravenously. Parenteral feeding requires the frequent changing of giving sets which is simplified by the presence of a stopcock. The second portal of the stopcock should be sealed with a sterile bung or cap if not in use.

Other items which may be required.
Thread stitch on a cutting needle — stitching the catheter in place has the merit of making it more difficult for the restless patient to displace the catheter, as well as permitting greater freedom of movement; it minimises sliding of the catheter in and out of the wound, thus

decreasing the chance of infection; and needs only a small dressing over the wound.

A 20ml syringe filled with saline. Some people prefer to use a syringe on the end of the introducing needle when probing for 'hidden' veins like the internal juglar and the subclavian, feeling that it is easier to locate the vein in this way. This method cannot be used with catheters such as the Drum Cartridge Catheter where the catheter cannot be detached from the needle.

After the catheter has been inserted successfully, the stilette is withdrawn, the catheter joined to the giving set via the two-way stopcock, and the drip is allowed to run freely for a second or two before being adjusted to a slow rate.

Adjustment and fixation

The length of the catheter inside the vein, or the position of the tip of the catheter, may be estimated by using the discarded stilette as a guide. The position of the catheter is adjusted if necessary. The needle is then withdrawn and its guard fixed in place, or removed altogether if this is possible. Pressure is applied to the area where appropriate, as soon as the needle is withdrawn. If the catheter is to be stitched in place, the stitch is inserted and tied round catheter where it passes through the skin, and the thread then *laced* along the catheter with a half knot every crossing, tied gently but firmly. If the thread is simply knotted round the catheter in one place, it will probably be tight enough to kink the catheter but not tight enough to prevent it from being pulled out. This is particularly likely with some of the softer catheters. Lacing provides adequate friction without kinking. A small elastoplast dressing may then be placed over the wound. If pressure is maintained over the venepuncture site from the time the needle is withdrawn until the dressing is applied, there will usually be minimal leakage from the wound.

If the catheter is not stitched in place, some form of adhesive strapping will be required to retain the catheter in place.

The Venous Pressure Manometer

The venous pressure manometer is made up of a drip set a manometer

The Measurement of Venous Pressure

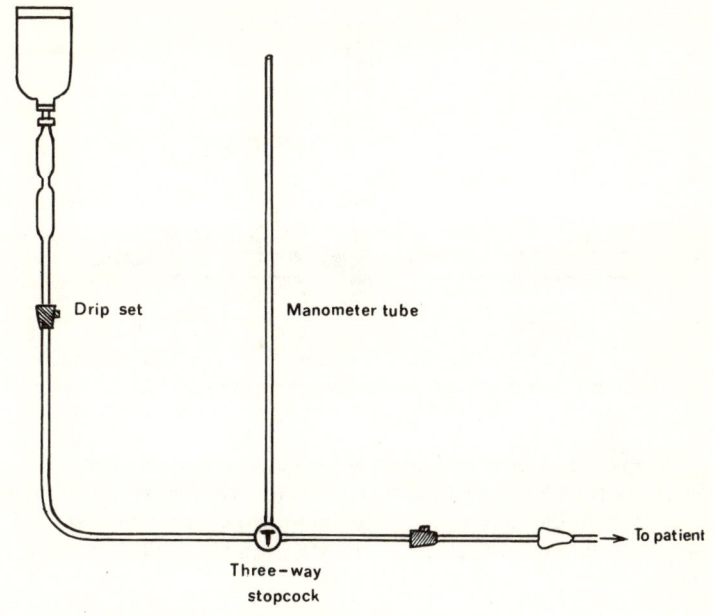

Fig. 5.4 Venous Pressure Manometer set.

When the CVP is read, the drip set is shut off from the patient and the manometer is brought into use by means of the stopcock or tap.

Taking a CVP reading

As with arterial pressure measurement, venous pressure readings should be taken 'on the fall'. This means that the manometer tubing must be full, and it is usual to refill it as soon as a reading has been taken, in preparation for the next observation. Obviously the manometer must be filled prior to the first reading; a height of 25–30 cms should be adequate. Once the pressure has been established, the manometer need be filled only 5–10 cms above this level to avoid infusing an unnecessary amount of fluid every time a reading is taken.

Check that the zero of the measuring scale is at the level of the sternal notch or whichever reference point is used, and that the manometer tubing is filled. Turn the tap so that the manometer is connected to the patient.

The fluid level in the manometer tube will fall quite rapidly for a few cms. As the level approaches the patient's CVP, the smooth fall slows down and becomes interrupted by pauses. Eventually the level falls no

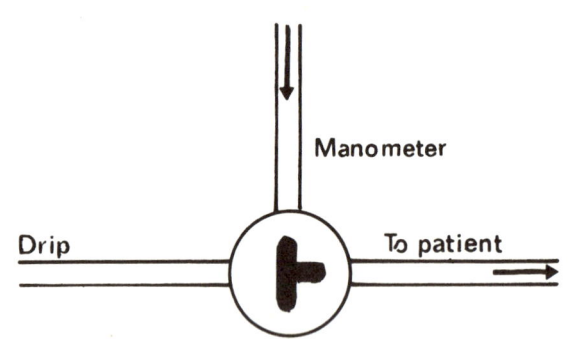

Fig. 5.5 The tap handles indicate the connections available — in this example, between the manometer and the patient.

more, merely swinging up and down as the patient breathes. The height of the fluid level in cms at this moment, measured in cms of saline is the pressure in the central great veins and the right atrium — the CVP.

Now turn the tap so that the manometer can be re-filled from the drip set.

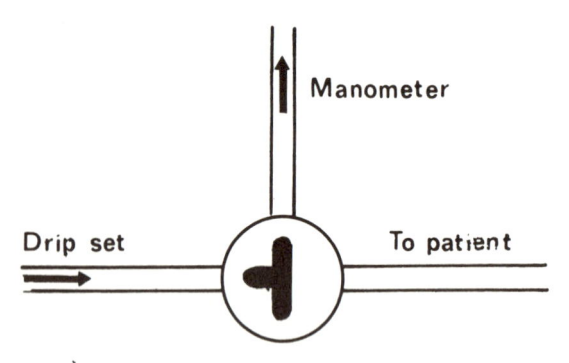

Fig. 5.6 The tap handle indicates the direction of flow — from the drip set to the manometer tube.

It is reasonable to speed up this process by increasing the drip rate for a second or two. Then return the tap to the drip-to-patient position and restore the slow rate of infusion.

What is the CVP?

The CVP measured with a simple saline manometer is the mean value of the pressure in the central great veins and the right atrium.

The Measurement of Venous Pressure

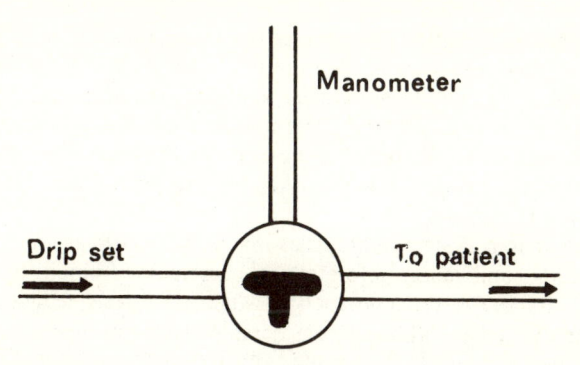

Fig. 5.7 The direction of flow is from the drip set to the patient.

A low CVP indicates   a low blood volume (hypovolaemia) or

an increase in the capacity of the circulatory system.

A high CVP indicates   an inefficient cardiac pump in the presence of a normal blood volume or

an excessive circulating blood volume (hypervolaemia)

A CVP within the normal range *implies* that the blood volume is normal and that the heart is able to pump out the blood supplied to it.

The word implies is used because as we have already seen,

1) there may be a raised left atrial pressure which is not revealed by right atrial pressure monitoring.
2) hypovolaemia may exist in the presence of a CVP which is within the normal range, owing to the ability of the body to compensate for acute blood or fluid loss.

CVP readings following acute blood loss

Immediately following acute blood loss, the venous return to the heart, the right atrial pressure and the output from both ventricles is reduced. The body responds in such a way so as to restore the cardiac output to as near normal levels as possible.

1) Sympathetic activity stimulates the myocardial fibres to shorten more than usual when they contract. Although the fall in right atrial pressure reduces ventricular filling, the heart can expel the smaller volume of blood presented to it efficiently because it can contract down further than normal. At the same time, the heart rate is increased. These measures tend to restore the cardiac output towards normal.
2) The venous system contains as much as 50–70% of the total blood volume, and can therefore act as a reservoir of blood. Sympathetic activity causes venoconstriction which effectively reduces the capacity of the circulation. A considerable volume of blood from this venous reservoir is thus made available to boost the venous return to the heart, and the CVP may rise a little, depending on the original volume of blood lost. Remember that although the total volume of blood available has been reduced, the volume it has to fill has also been diminished.
3) If the volume of blood lost exceeds that which can be brought into the circulation by venoconstriction, the circulating blood volume becomes insufficient even for the reduced capacity of the circulation. The pressure in the right atrium falls again, as indicated by the CVP, and peripheral perfusion becomes inadequate. Arteriolar constriction occurs to divert blood to vital tissues from others such as the skin and splanchnic organs. The reduction in peripheral perfusion leads to a fall in tissue capillary pressure below that of the osmotic pressure of the plasma proteins, and water passes into the capillaries from the interstitial fluid. It has been shown that 500–700 ml of fluid may enter this way into the circulation within 5 minutes following a massive acute haemorrhage. Although the CVP is low, the arterial blood pressure is frequently maintained within normal limits at this stage, due to the effects of venous and arteriolar constriction, the increased myocardial efficiency and the rise in heart rate.

If the loss of blood continues however, the compensatory mechanisms are eventually exhausted and the arterial blood pressure falls.

It can be seen that arterial pressure and CVP readings *on their own* can be misleading, since the initial response of the body to acute blood or fluid loss is increased cardiac efficiency, a near normal cardiac output and a CVP which may well be within normal limits. Where there is suspicion of a reduction in circulating blood volume, the patient should be transfused with the appropriate fluid until the CVP rises to the upper limit of normal. The response to transfusion will confirm the presence of hypovolaemia; the rising CVP is accompanied by a rise in blood pressure, a fall in pulse rate and clinical evidence of an improved peripheral circulation — warm, pink peripheries, well-filled veins and an increased urinary output.

In the presence of myocardial disease, CVP readings must always be assessed with care and in conjunction with the clinical state of the patient, as well as with the history of events leading up to the current state. In the normal heart, it may be assumed that both ventricles are working efficiently; the presence of myocardial makes that assumption a dangerous one since the CVP reading reflects only the efficiency of the right ventricle.

6

Some Drugs Used in Intensive Care

The list of drugs in common use on page 67 deliberately includes some trade names. Although we all try to conform to the concept of using approved or official names, the fact remains that quite a lot of us concerned with the prescribing and administration of drugs still use trade names, if only because the trade name of a drug on an ampule, vial or box is printed in larger letters than the approved or official name and is thus more easily identified. Furthermore, many trade names are frequently easier to remember than the official ones, and a glance at any drug cupboard will confirm that many of the contents stacked inside have their trade names not their official names re-written on the sides of the boxes.

Numbers and Doses. Many people are not entirely at ease with numbers, and I therefore make no apology to those who do not share this problem for the next few paragraphs.

Some of the difficulties arise because of incomplete understanding of the principles of the decimal system. Others occur because a sort of conventional shorthand is often employed. I have come across not a few people who thought that 0.35 mg was a larger quantity than 0.5 mg until the latter was re-written 0.50 mg.

The decimal system is based on the number ten (Latin decem — 10) and a decimal point is used to separate FRACTIONS (on the right of the point) from WHOLE NUMBERS (on the left). The fractions commonly used are tenths, hundredths and thousandths, and the size of the fraction is indicated by the position of the decimal point. Whole numbers are treated in the same way

one tenth is written 0.1
one hundreth is written 0.01
one thousandth is written 0.001

The same principle applies to whole numbers:

$$1.0$$
$$10.0$$
$$100.0$$
$$1000.0$$

If a decimal figure is multiplied by 10, the decimal point is simply moved one place, to the right,

$$0.10 \times 10 = 01.0$$
$$0.01 \times 10 = 00.1$$

If a decimal figure is divided by 10, the decimal point is moved one place to the left,

$$0.10 \div 10 = .010$$

Multiplication or division by 100 moves the decimal point two places, and by 1000, three places.

There are 1000 milligrams (1000 mg) in 1 gram (1 g)

1 mg is therefore one thousandth of a gram and can be written 0.00	
10 mg can be written 0.010 g	
35 mg	0.035 g
100 mg	0.100 g — usually abbreviated to 0.1 g
500 mg	0.500 g — usually abbreviated to 0.5 g
1000 mg	1.000 g — usually abbreviated to 1.0 g

Where whole numbers only are employed, the noughts on the right of the decimal point are frequently omitted. This is often done with fractions too,

e.g. 1 g instead of 1.0 g
10 mg instead of 10.0 mg
0.5 g instead of 0.50 g
0.6 mg instead of 0.60 mg.

It is unforgivable however to omit a nought on the *left* hand side of the decimal point when fractions are involved,

e.g. .6 mg instead of 0.6 mg
.5 g instead of 0.5 g

Errors are more than possible when prescriptions involving fractions are written in such a way. Errors in both prescribing and administration are likely when very small quantities are required, as in paediatrics.

e.g. digoxin 0.0125 mg
atropine 0.0018 mg

In such circumstances, it may well be safer to use the next *range* of units — in this case, micrograms — in order to avoid the necessity for so many decimal places. There are 1000 micrograms (mcg) in 1 mg, so to convert the mg dose to mcg, the number must be multiplied by 1000. There are three noughts in 1000 so the decimal point is moved three places to the right. Noughts are added or removed as necessary.

digoxin 0.0125 mg x 1000 = 12.5 mcg

atropine 0.0018 mg x 1000 = 1.8 mcg

atropine 0.6 mg x 1000 = 600.0 mcg

Units in common use are the kilogram
the gram
the milligram
the microgram

1 kilogram	=	1000 grams
1 gram	=	1000 milligrams
1 milligram	=	1000 micrograms

Units of *volume* are derived from units of length,

e.g. centimetre cubed cm^3 The alternative description — cubic centimetre — provides the familiar abbreviation cc.

An International system of units has been established and one result has been the disappearance of some familiar names. The term *Litre* has however been officially retained and millilitres (ml) are acceptable as fractions of a litre. The abbreviation for cubic centimetre — cc — is now officially obsolete. Examples of symbols which can be seen are:

kilogram	— official symbol kg	Variants — Kg, kilo
gram	— g	— gm, gms, grammes
milligram	— mg	— mgm
microgram	— μg (μ the Greek letter m, pronounced mew)	— mcg — but in prescriptions, the unit should be written in full, not abbreviated to mcg.

Some Drugs Used in Intensive Care

Solutions

Concentration, strength, tonicity and dilution are all terms used to describe solutions. They indicate

> how much of a substance is present in a solution.

The terms may be used in various ways:

> 'make a concentrated solution of . . .
> well-diluted
> a solution of high concentration . . .
> the strength of a solution . . .
> the concentration of the solution is . . .
> a hypertonic solution . . .'

> and so on.

Concentration is defined as

> the quantity of a substance present in a unit of *weight*
> or the quantity of a substance present in a unit of *volume*

> for example — so much of a substance in 100 grams of water
> or — so much of a substance in 1 litre of water

The quantity of the substance can be expressed in any convenient units but *weight* is commonly employed,

> e.g. the concentration of salt in sea water is 3.6 grams in 100 grams.

In this example, the concentration is defined in terms of *weight per weight*. Alternatively, using the definition of *weight per volume*,

> the concentration of atropine in water for injection is 0.6 mg per ml.

Concentrations are often described in terms of weight per volume with no units mentioned, and under those circumstances, by convention, the units involved are *grams per ml*.

> Abbreviation is common — W/V for weight per volume
> W/W for weight per weight

It may be convenient to use 100 ml rather than 1 ml as the unit of volume. Concentration then becomes *Percentage weight per volume*,

> e.g. the concentration of a solution of X in water is 0.5 grams % W/V

> i.e. 0.5 grams (W) per
> 100 ml (V)

Again, if no units are mentioned, a % W/V concentration implies grams per 100 ml. Not infrequently, the description W/V is omitted, and the solution is described only as a percentage solution, e.g.

>Brietal 1%, lignocaine 2%   and so on.

These solutions are in fact % W/V solutions and the units involved are grams/100 ml.

We must know the actual quantity of a drug we are giving. This is no problem where the drug is presented as the prescribed amount,

>e.g. Fentazin   5 mg
>
>Omnopon   20 mg.

Both these drugs come in ampules of 1 ml which contain the amounts mentioned above. Where a variable quantity of a drug is required, as in the induction of anaesthesia with thiopentone for example, the drug is provided in a suitable concentration and the actual quantity administered is calculated from the concentration,

e.g. thiopentone 2.5%

A patient has been given 16 ml of the 2.5% solution.
2.5% is 2.5 grams per 100 ml

$$= 2.5 \times 1000 \text{ mg per 100 ml}$$

$$= 2.5 \times \frac{1000}{100} \text{ mg per ml}$$

$$= 25 \text{ mg/ml}$$

so the patient has been given 16 × 25 mg

$$= 400 \text{ mg}$$

Of course there is no need to use the long calculation every time — it should be clear from the example above that a % concentration is easily converted into mg/ml by multiplying by 10 $\left(\frac{1000}{100} = 10\right)$

>thus   1% Brietal is 10 mg/ml
>2% Lignocaine is 20 mg/ml
>0.5% lignocaine is 5 mg/ml   and so on.

Some Drugs Used in Intensive Care

Adrenaline
Aminophylline
Ampicillin (Penbritin)
Atropine

Bupivacaine (Marcaine)

Calcium chloride
Carbenicillin (Pyopen)
Cephaloridine (Cephorin)
Caphalothin (Keflex)
Chloramphenicol

Cortisol (Hydrocortisone)
Dexamethasone
Diazepam (Valium)
Digoxin
Droperidol
Doxapram (Dopram)

Ephedrine

Fentanyl (Sublimaze)
Flucloxacillin
Frusemide (Lasix)

Gentamycin
Glucagon

Isoprenaline

Ketamine (Ketalar)

Lignocaine (Xylocaine)

Mannitol (Osmitrol)
Methadone (Physeptone)
Methohexitone (Brietal)
Methoxamine (Vasoxine)
Methylamphetamine (Methedrine)
Metoclopramide (Maxalon)
Morphine

Nalorphine (Lethidrone)
Neostigmine (Prostigmine)
Nikethamide (Coramine)
Noradrenaline (Levophed)

Pancuronium (Pavulon)
Penicillin
Pentazocine (Fortral)
Pentolinium (Ansolysen)
Perphenzine (Fentazin)
Pethidine
Phenobarbitone
Phenoperidine
Phentolamine (Rogitine)
Phenytoin   (Epanutin)
Practolol

Procaineamide
Propranolol   (Inderal)
Pyridostigmine (Mestinon)

Salbutamol
Sodium bicarbonate
Sodium nitroprusside
Streptomycin
Strophanthin G

Suxemethonium (Anectine)

Tetracycline
Thiopentone
Trimetaphan (Arfonad)
Trimethoprim
Tubocurarine

ADRENALINE

Adrenaline stimulates the *alpha* receptors of the sympathetic nervous system producing peripheral vasoconstriction, and the *beta* receptors producing an increase in pulse rate and myocardial contractility. It is used in the treatment of cardiac arrest to stimulate the heart. Although it produces *vasodilatation* in *muscle,* the vasoconstrictor action tends to predominate so that the blood pressure remains within the normal range and coronary perfusion is not impaired.

Adrenaline also relaxes smooth muscle of the bronchi and is therefore useful in the treatment of bronchospasm. It is used with local anaesthetics for its vasoconstrictor properties which decrease the rate of absorption of the anaesthetic agent. It is also used in the treatment of angioneurotic oedema and other allergic conditions.

1) Brown ampule of 1 ml containing 1 in 1000 adrenaline (1 mg/ml)
2) Clear ampule of 10 ml containing 1 in 10,000 adrenaline (0.1 mg/ml).

Aminophylline

Aminophylline relaxes smooth muscle, especially that of the bronchial tree. It also stimulates the myocardium and is a mild central nervous stimulant.

It is used in the treatment of asthma and acute left ventricular failure and is given by *slow* intravenous injection in these cases, since rapid injection may cause cardiac arrest. It also produces renel vasodilatation and can be used to increase the diuretic response to frusemide.

Aminophylline suppositories are useful in the treatment of chronic bronchospasm.

1) Ampules of 10 ml containing 250 mg
2) Tablets of 100 mg and suppositories of 360 mg.

Ampicillin (Penbritin)

A general purpose broad spectrum antibiotic. Remarkably free from toxic effects except in those patients who are sensitive to penicillin derivatives. Resistant organisms are becoming more common.

An unstable substance which must be made up before use.

Vials of dry powder (Penbritin – Beecham laboratories) containing 100, 250 or 500 mg.

Atropine

Atropine blocks the action of acetylcholine on the parasympathetic nervous system and so causes:-

1) Tachycardia
2) Drying of secretions in the mouth, gut and tracheobronchial tree
3) Relaxation of the smooth muscle of the gut
4) Dilatation of the pupil (in large doses – over 2.0 mg).

The main uses of atropine are:-
   a) to abolish bradycardia induced by vagal stimulation. It is *not* effective in bradycardia due to heart block or digitalis overdose.
   b) As premedication to reduce secretions in the tracheobronchial tree and to reduce the effects of vagal stimulation induced during intubation and surgery.
   c) To counteract the parasympathetic effects of neostigmine, which is used to reverse muscle relaxants and in the treatment of Myasthenia Gravis.
   d) As eye drops to dilate the pupil for a long period, e.g. in the management of iritis.

   1 ml ampule of Atropine Sulphate containing 0.6 mg/ml (600 mcg – micrograms – per ml).

Bupivacaine (Marcaine)

Bupivacaine is a local analgesic similar to lignocaine but with a much longer duration of action – 4 to 8 hours. It also differs from lignocaine in that

   it does not have such marked sedative and anti-dysrhythmic properties
   it does not spread so well in tissues planes
   it produces only slight vasoconstriction.

It is commonly combined with adrenaline to produce long-acting analgesia, e.g. to control the pain of fractured ribs by continuous epidural block.

   10 ml Ampules containing 0.5% solution (5 mg/ml) plain, or with adrenaline 1 in 200,000
   0.25% solution (2.5 mg/ml) plain, or with adrenaline 1 in 400,000.

Calcium Chloride

Calcium ions improve the force of contraction of any muscle, especially cardiac muscle. Calcium chloride is therefore often used in emergency situations to stimulate a failing heart for short periods.

Stored blood contains more potassium ions in the serum than normal. A high serum potassium level causes weak myocardial contractions. Calcium chloride is therefore given during massive or rapid blood transfusion to improve myocardial contraction and to counteract the effects due to hyperkalaemia.

Ampules of 10 ml Calcium Chloride 1%
10 ml Calcium Gluconate 10%.

Carbenicillin (Pyopen)

A synthetic antibiotic of the penicillin group. One of the few antibiotics effective against Pseudomonas although resistant strains are becoming more common. Penicillin sensitivity is a contra-indication to its use.

Intramuscular injection is very painful, so the drug should be given mixed with lignocaine.

Cephaloridine (Cephorin)

One of the cephalosporin group of antibiotics. A broad spectrum antibiotic to which, at present, only a few organisms are resistant. It has been known to cause renal failure, especially when used in conjunction with frusemide. It must be given parenterally as it is not absorbed by mouth.

Cephalothin (Keflin)

Another of the cephalosporin group of antibiotics. A broad spectrum antibiotic to which most organisms are still sensitive. Few side effects. Like cephaloridine, it is not absorbed by mouth.

Chloramphenicol (Chloromycetin)

A very effective effective broad spectrum antibiotic. Unfortunately it causes bone marrow depression, and occasionally aplastic anaemia so its use is somewhat restricted. It is the drug of choice for severe Haemophilus influenzae infections and typhoid fever, and is useful as a topical antiobiotic, e.g. Chloramphenicol eye ointment.

Cortisol (Hydrocortisone)

A naturally occurring steroid hormone produced by the adrenal cortex. The hormone is commonly referred to as hydrocortisone but levels in the blood are referred to as blood cortisol levels. Previously used in large doses to prevent inflammatory reactions; the synthetic hormones now available, e.g. dexamethasone, prednisolone, are preferred to cortisol as they do not interfere with the measurement of the cortisol produced by the patient.

Cortisol (Hydrocortisone) is still used to treat patients who have collapsed due to adrenocortical insufficiency in the form of the soluable hydrocortisone sodium succinate. It has a potent effect on the cardiovascular system

> increasing cardiac output,
> decreasing capillary permeability,
> restoring the vasomotor response to normal.

Efcortelan Soluble (Glaxo) Hydrocortisone Sodium Succinate
Solu-Cortef (Up-john) Hydrocortisone Sodium Succinate

as dry powder in vials, containing 100 mg, supplied with 2 ml water.

Dexamethasone (Decadron, Oradexon)

A potent synthetic steroid used to reduce inflammatory reactions. It is very useful in the treatment of cerebral oedema and aspiration pneumonitis (Mendelson's syndrome). It may produce dramatic improvement in patients with cerebral oedema due to cerebral matastases and other cerebral tumours.

Decadron   2 ml ampule containing 4 mg/ml

Oradexon   1 ml ampule containing 5 mg/ml.

Diazepam (Valium)

A benzdiazepine. A very effective tranquillizer, which can be given intravenously, intramuscularly or orally. It can produce unconsciousness if given rapidly I/V. It does *not* give any *analgesia* so should not be used alone in the management of the patient in pain. Diazepam causes only slight respiratory depression but will certainly produce respiratory failure and coma in the patient who is already in severe respiratory distress — these patients are often very agitated and restless because of hypoxia, and treatment should be aimed at improving oxygenation and ventilation rather than sedation.

Diazepam decreases myocardial irritability and is therefore popular for cardioversion. In large doses it is used in the treatment of status epilepticus and toxaemia of pregnancy. Diazepam often causes pain when given intravenously so it should be given slowly, preferably into a fast-running drip. It should *not* be diluted in *small* volumes of fluid as the drug will precipitate out of its polythene glycol solvent. Lignocaine 2 ml of 2% can be given intravenously before diazepam is administered to reduce the pain of injection.

Valium (Roche)   Brown ampule of 2 ml containing 5 mg/ml

Also capsules and tablet and syrups of varying strengths.

Digoxin (Lanoxin)

Digoxin is the most commonly used of the cardiac glycosides. Its effects are
 a) An increase in the force of contraction of the myocardium
 b) Depression of the conduction mechanisms of the heart — slowing the rate and eventually producing complete heart block.
 c) An increase in myocardial excitability — so that the threshold for dysrhythmia is lowered.
 d) Stimulation of the vagus — which causes bradycardia.

The actions of digoxin are potentiated by a low serum potassium and a high serum calcium. Digoxin is excreted in the urine so the dose has to be reduced in patients with renal failure. The elderly respond in the same way as other patients but excrete the drug more slowly and so require smaller doses. Digoxin is absorbed erractically when given intramuscularly. If oral administration is contraindicated, digoxin should be given intravenously via a mini-dripper, diluted in 50—120 ml of fluid.

Digoxin is used in the treatment of atrial fibrillation, since it results in a degree of heart block which will produce an effective ventricular rate (about 80) in the presence of a very high atrial rate (about 500). It is also useful in the treatment of any form of heart failure, though at the risk of producing dysrhythmias. The therapeutic dose is close to the toxic dose, so blood levels are often measured to control dosage. Toxic effects (ventricular ectopics, coupled beats and ventricular tachycardia) are best treated with beta adrenergic blocking agents, e.g. practolol, and stopping the digoxin.

2 ml ampule containing 0.5 mg (0.25 mg/ml)
Tablets of 0.25 mg.

Doxapram (Dopram)

A respiratory stimulant, given as an intravenous drip, whose rate must be very carefully controlled (e.g. by a Mini-drip). It may be useful in avoiding artificial ventilation in chronic bronchitis with acute-on-chronic respiratory failure. It may also be useful in weaning patients with chronic respiratory failure off ventilators.

500 ml of 5% Dextrose containing Doxapram 2 mg/ml (total amount in 500 ml—1 gram).

Droperidol (Droleptan)

Droperidol is a butyrophenone. The butyrophenones are related to the phenothiazines. Droperidol is a potent tranquillizer and anti-emetic. It also has an alpha-adrenergic blocking action and so may be used to lower the blood pressure. (Stimulation of the alpha-receptors produces vasoconstriction so blocking this action leads to vasodilatation and a fall in blood pressure). Droperidol is mainly used as a tranquilliser, often in conjunction with potent analgesics such as phenoperidine to produce the state known as Neuroleptanalgesia. One major problem with droperidol is that although the patients appear tranquil at the time, afterwards they may complain that they were in fact very frightened. Droperidol with or without phenoperidine has virtually no effect on the electroencephalogram, which may be useful in intensive care situations.

2 ml ampule containing 5 mg/ml
Tablets of 10 mg.

Ephedrine

Ephedrine is a synthetic drug, related chemically to adrenaline. It raises the blood pressure mainly by increasing heart rate and myocardial contractility, although it also causes some peripheral vasoconstriction.

Ephedrine is also useful as a bronchodilator in patients with bronchospasm. It has also been used in the treatment of Myasthenia Gravis as it improves neuro-muscular conduction.

2 ml ampule containing 30 mg

Fentanyl (Sublimaze)

This is a synthetic analgesic drug derived from pethidine, and very similar to phenoperidine. Like phenoperidine it has virtually no effect on the cardiovascular system. The only significant difference between fentanyl and phenoperidine is in duration of action — 20 minutes when given intravenously for fentanyl compared with 45 minutes for phenoperidine.

2 ml ampule containing 0.05 mg/ml	total amount in ampule 0.1 mg
10 ml ampule	" " " " 0.5 mg.

Flucloxacillin (Floxapen)

A synthetic antibiotic of the penicillin group. It is mainly used for the treatment of infections due to gram-positive organisms, resistant to other antibiotics, especially Staph. aureus. May be given orally or by injection.

Frusemide (Lasix)

A powerful diuretic which acts by preventing the kidney from reabsorbing sodium and potassium and therefore the water which goes with these ions. The loss of potassium is such that potassium supplements must be given either orally or intravenously during frusemide therapy. It may precipitate an attack of gout and cause hyperglycaemia. Large doses of up to 1 g may be used in certain conditions, but the normal dose is 20–80 mg.

Brown ampule of 2 ml containing 20 mg.

Gentamycin

A broad spectrum antibiotic, usually reserved for use against Pseudomonas and Proteus which are resistent to most antibiotics. It is excreted solely by the kidneys. The major risks in its use are renal damage and ototoxicity. Blood levels should always be measured since the therapeutic index is very low. It must be given by injection as it is poorly absorbed from the gastrointestinal tract.

2 ml ampule containing 40 mg.

Glucagon

Glucagon is the hormone secreted by the alpha cells of the Islets of Langerhans in the pancreas (insulin is secreted by the beta cells). Glucagon *raises* the blood sugar by releasing glucose from glycogen in the liver. It has also been found to have a direct inotropic action on the myocardium, i.e. it increases the force of contraction. This stimulant action is independent of the action of digitalis and sympathomimetic drugs, so it is a useful drug in emergency situations. It will also combat the myocardial depression produced by propranalol; propranalol acts by blocking the sympathetic beta receptors but glucagon acts directly on the myocardial fibres, thus by-passing the receptor block, to increase the heart rate and improve the force of contraction.

1 ml Ampule containing 1 mg glucagon powder together with a 1 ml ampule of water

10 ml Ampule containing 10 mg glucagon powder together with a 10 ml ampule of water.

Isoprenaline

A catechol amine, chemically very similar to adrenaline. It is a powerful cardiac stimulant, increasing both the heart rate (chronotrophic action) and the force of contraction (inotropic action), and therefore myocardial oxygen consumption. This makes it a dangerous drug in the presence of myocardial infarction. If the myocardial blood supply is precarious due to infarction it is likely that the increased demand for oxygen produced by the effects of isoprenaline cannot be satisfied, and a further number of cells may die. Isoprenaline, may therefore *increase the extent* of a myocradial infarct. It also produces peripheral vasodilatation by relaxing smooth muscle so it may cause a fall in blood pressure. It is usually given via a Mini-dripper under E.C.G. control.

It is also used in the treatment of bronchospasm, where it is administered topically to the bronchial tree via an inhaler.

Overdosage results in tachycardia and ventricular dysrhythmias.

Ampule of 1 ml containing 0.2 mg

" 5 ml containing 1.0 mg.

Ketamine (Ketalar, Ketaject)

Ketamine is a dissociative anaesthetic agent which can be given either intravenously or intramuscularly. Pharyngeal and laryngeal reflexes usually remain unaffected so that the patient can maintain his own airway. It is therefore very useful for the patient with airway problems, e.g. from burns. It is also a cardiovascular stimulant producing a rise in blood pressure and pulse rate, so it can be useful for the induction of anaesthesia in bad-risk patients but it is usually avoided in hypertensive patients.

The main disadvantage of ketamine is the occurrence of hallucinations and nightmares during arousal; these usually only occur in adults and can be considerably reduced by giving diazepam at the end of the procedure, or a sedative as premedication. Patients recovering from ketamine anaesthesia should be left completely undisturbed and not stimulated in any way in order to reduce the incidence of hallucinations. The drug has considerable analgesic properties.

Vials of 10 ml containing 50 mg/ml
"   10 ml   "   100 mg/ml.

Lignocaine (Xylocaine)

Lignocaine is mainly used as a local analgesic agent. It also reduces the excitability of the myocardium and is of considerable value in the treatment of ventricular dysrhythmias. It depresses atrio-ventricular conduction, and in high doses it will reduce myocardial contraction and cause cerebral convulsions. There are many different concentrations available. Make sure that the solutions for intravenous use do not contain adrenaline or preservative.

Although very large doses or a temporary high blood level produced by injecting a strong solution too rapidly will produce convulsions, lignocaine does possess a sedative effect when used in smaller doses and has been used for the treatment of status epilepticus.

Various ampules of 1, 2, 5, 10, 20 and 30 ml whose concentrations range from 0.5 to 2%, both with and without adrenaline. Maximum dose of the drug used as a bolus injection − 200 mg.

Mannitol (Osmitrol)

Mannitol is chemically similar to glucose and fructose, but it is not metabolised by the body and is excreted unchanged in the urine. It therefore produces an *osmotic diuresis*. Mannitol is given as a 10% or 20% solution. These solutions are hypertonic and the giving set should be changed or flushed with an isotonic electrolyte solution before giving blood, otherwise the red cells will be damaged by the hypertonic solution. Crystals may form if the solution is allowed to get cold but they redissolve if the bottle is warmed.

Methadone (Physeptone)

A synthetic analgesic similar to morphine. Like morphine it produces

    a) Analgesia
    b) Respiratory depression
    c) Depression of the cough reflex
    d) Nausea and vomiting
    e) Orthostatic hypotension
    f) Addiction

The chief difference between methadone and morphine is that the duration of action is less with methadone — 2 hours as opposed to 4 hours when given intramuscularly. Methadone also produces less euphoria. It is used mainly if analgesia is required when it is essential to assess the mental state of the patient. It is the only opiate which may be given in a maintainance dose to a registered addict by an ordinary doctor; it is also used in the withdrawal treatment of opiate addiction.

    Ampule of 1 ml containing 10 mg

    Also tablets and linctus.

Methohexitone (Brietal)

A short-acting barbiturate similar to thiopentone used for the induction of anaesthesia. The recovery time is shorter than that for thiopentone and so it is often used for short anaesthetics, e.g. for bronchoscopy.

    Ampules, vials and bottles of varying capacity to be made up to a 1% solution (10 mg/ml). Concentrations of 2% are also available.

    Average induction dose — 100 mg, i.e. 10 ml of the 1% solution.

Methylamphetamine (Methedrine)

A synthetic drug, with similar effects to adrenaline. It raises the blood pressure mainly by increasing heart rate and myocardial contractility, although it also causes peripheral vasoconstriction. It is probably the best vasopressor drug to use if the pulse is slow. Like all amphetamines it is a central nervous stimulant and so wakes patients up. As it has been abused by amphetamine addicts it is no longer manufactured but existing stocks may last a long time.

Ampule of 1 ml containing 20 mg

1.5 ml containing 30 mg.

Metoclopramide (Maxolon)

An anti-emetic drug which acts by increasing gastric emptying and also to a lesser degree directly on the central nervous system. This action on the stomach is abolished by atropine. Unlike most anti-emetics it does not cause much drowsiness. It is also effective in controlling hiccough and is used by radiologists to speed up Barium follow-throughs. It is also used prior to emergency anaesthesia to help empty the stomach — but remember that this action is lost as soon as a premedication containing atropine is given. The anti-emetic effect is *not* strong enough to overcome vomiting caused by opiates.

Ampule of 2 ml containing 10 mg

Also tablets and syrup.

Morphine

One of the oldest and most effective of the analgesic agents, which also has a marked euphoric action. It is used as the standard with which the newer analgesic agents are compared.

The important side effects of morphine are

a) Respiratory depression — this is the main factor in limiting the dose which can safely be given, but if the patient is being ventilated artificially, large doses can be given safely, e.g. during anaesthesia, as much as 100 mg in 1 hour. Morphine is employed for its respiratory depressant effects to control patients on ventilators.
The respiratory depressant effect can be antagonised by nalorphine.
b) Depression of the cough reflex.
c) Nausea and vomiting. It is a good idea to give an anti-emetic with morphine initially to control nausea and vomiting, but tolerance to this side effect develops rapidly. If a phenothiazine is used as an

Some Drugs Used in Intensive Care

anti-emetic, hypotension may occur, and the respiratory depressant effect of the morphine is potentiated.

d) Construction of smooth muscle. Morphine may be poorly tolerated by some asthmatics as it may make their bronchospasm worse. Constriction of the smooth muscle of the bowel causes constipation, and may also cause the breakdown of large bowel anastomoses or perforation of obstructed bowel. Morphine should be avoided in these situations. Smooth muscle constriction produces the characteristic pin-point pupils; morphine should not be used if pupil signs are essential in the assessment of the patient, e.g. following head injury.

e) Release of histamine. This may cause hypotension but it usually only results in itching, especially of the nose.

f) Addiction. This is unlikely provided the patient is emotionally stable to begin with. Most patients are only too glad to stop the drug once the clinical indication has passed. It is cruel to withhold morphine from a patient in pain for fear that they may become addicted.

Ampules containing 8, 10, 15 and 20 mg/ml.

Nalorphine (Lethidrone)

Nalorphine is an opiate derivative which is a moderate analgesic in its own right. It acts as a competitive inhibitor of morphine and is therefore used to antagonise the respiratory depressant effects of morphine and its derivatives; at the same time it also antagonises the analgesic effect. Mixtures of opiates and nalorphine have been tried in order to produce an analgesic with less respiratory depression, but these have not proved successful since the analgesia becomes much less effective.

Ampule of 1 ml containing 10 mg.

Neostigmine (Prostigmine)

Neostigmine is an anti-cholinesterase. Cholinesterase breaks down acetylcholine, so that preventing this action by administering an anticholinesterase leads to an *increase* in the body's acetylcholine.

The effects of *acetylcholine* can be classified as a) muscarinic
b) nicotinic

The *muscarinic* effects are those associated with parasympathetic activity and include

a) increased production of saliva, sweat, bronchial, gastric and intestinal secretions
b) increased activity of the gut
c) constriction of the pupil
d) bradycardia

These effects are antagonised by atropine.

The *nicotinic* effects are those which occur at the neuromuscular junction, i.e. contraction of striated muscle.

These effects are antagonised by curate and other non-depolarising muscle relaxants.

The non-depolarising muscle relaxants produce their antagonistic effect (i.e. paralysis) by preventing acetylcholine gaining access to the receptors on the muscle end-plate because they are present in greater concentration. This action is called competitive inhibition. A drug such as neostigmine which produces an increase in the amount of acetylcholine can therefore be used to reverse this inhibition.

Too much neostigmine will impede the action of cholinesterase to such an extent that acetylcholine is continuously present to stimulate the muscle fibres – in other words, neostigmine can itself produce muscle paralysis. This situation is unlikely to occur following the reversal of muscle relaxants in anaesthesia, provided that not more than 5 mg of neostigmine is given, but it is not uncommon in Myasthenia Gravis where large doses are used in order to improve muscle power. The response to neostigmine in this disease is unpredictable and a previously effective dose can quickly become an overdose, producing the cholinergic crisis of myasthenia. The respiratory muscle paralysis associated with a cholinergic crisis may require swift intervention and mechanical ventilation.

Atropine is usually given with neostigmine in order to antagonise the muscarinic effects of acetylcholine when only the nicotinic effects on the muscle end-plate are required.

Nikethamide (Coramine)

Nikethamide is a central nervous stimulant producing arousal, hyperventilation, coughing, vomiting and in larger doses, convulsions. It has been used in the treatment of respiratory depression caused by drug overdose, and to encourage coughing in patients with sputum retention. Although it stimulates respiration it also increases oxygen consumption, so much of its usefulness is lost. It may still be used to produce a vigorous cough where a single bolus of sputum is causing trouble.

Ampule of 2 ml Nikethamide

Ampule of 2 ml Coramine (Ciba). Both are a 25% solution and the ampules contain 250 mg Nikethamide.

Nitrazepam (Mogadon)

A benzdiazepine, similar to diazepam (Valium) and used as a hypnotic. Like many hypnotics, it may well cause confusion and disorientation in the elderly. It can only be given orally.

Mogadon (Roche) white tables of 5 mg

purple and black capsules of 5 mg

syrup containing 5 mg in 5 ml.

Noradrenaline (Levophed)

A naturally occurring catechol amine with a predominant and stimulant effect. It causes a marked increase in blood pressure by stimulating peripheral vasoconstriction and myocardial contractility. The rise in blood pressure tends to produce a reflex slowing of the pulse. The peripheral vasoconstriction causes poor tissue perfusion and reduces renal blood flow drastically; noradrenaline is therefore hardly ever used alone now. If, however, it is given with phentolamine (an alpha blocking agent, which is also a potent myocardial stimulant) the potentially disadvantageous peripheral alpha effects are blocked and only the beta effects are seen — increased cardiac output and a rise in pulse rate, producing an increase in tissue perfusion. Noradrenaline/phentolamine mixtures thus have a similar action to isoprenaline, but are less likely to produce tachycardia and ventricular dysrhythmias. Like isoprenaline, noradrenaline increases myocardial oxygen consumption but to a lesser degree.

Noradrenaline is highly irritant and must always be diluted before use.

2 ml ampule — Levophed — containing noradrenaline tartrate 2 mg (= 1 mg/ml or 1 in 1000).

Pancuronium (Pavulon)

Pancuronium is a non-depolarising muscle relaxant, similar in action to tubocurarine. However, it has no ganglion-blocking action and so does not produce hypotension or paralytic ileus. The duration of action is similar to tubocurarine.

2 ml ampule containing 4 mg.

Penicillin

Penicillin is a bactericidal antibiotic mainly effective against streptococci and staphylococci, although most staphylococci in hospitals are now resistant to it. It is still the best antibiotic to use if the organisms are sensitive. Very few side effects occur, with the exception that some patients may become sensitized to it and death has followed subsequent administration. It is still used as routine antibiotic cover to prevent the development of subacute bacterial endocarditis due to strep. viridans in susceptible patients — i.e. those with rheumatic heart disease or congenital heart lesions.

Intramuscular injection of penicillin is painful. Intrathecally, only small doses should be given as large doses cause convulsions and death.

Pentazocine (Fortral)

This is a narcotic analgesic derived from nalorphine. It produces respiratory depression although this is not marked. Its chief advantage is that it is not a drug of addiction and is not controlled by the Dangerous Drugs Act. The disadvantage is that it is only a moderate analgesic, and disorientation is quite common as it is a potent hallucinogen. Pentazocine should not be used in the presence of myocardial infarction since it produces an increase in pulmonary artery pressure which could provoke heart failure.

Ampules of 1 and 2 ml containing 30 mg/ml

Also capsules, and tablets.

Pentolinium (Ansolysen)

Pentolinium is a ganglion-blocking drug which is used to produce hypotension. Like all ganglion blocking agents, the effect on the blood pressure can be altered by the posture of the patient. In young patients, the hypotension often results in a reflex adrenergic tachycardia which may need to be controlled with a beta-adrenergic blocking agent, e.g. propranalol. The autonomic ganglia of the gut are also blocked by pentolinium and paralytic ileus commonly occurs during its use. The ciliary ganglion of the eye is also effected so that patients receiving pentolinium have fixed, dilated pupils.

Vials of 10 ml containing a 0.5% solution, i.e. 5 mg/ml.

Perphenazine (Fentazin)

Perphenazine is a phenothiazine with a marked anti-emetic action. It also has sedative properties. A common side effect is hypotension, due to alpha adrenergic blockade producing peripheral vasodilatation. Overdose may cause extra-pyramidal signs such as tremor and oculo-gyric crises (rolling of the eyes). These look frightening but are not serious, and can be treated with intravenous atropine and stopping the perphenazine.

1 ml amoule containing 5 mg

Also tablets and syrup.

Pethidine

A synthetic analgesic similar to morphine. Like morphine it produces

1) Analgesia
2) Respiratory depression
3) Depression of the cough reflex
4) Nausea and vomiting
5) Hypotension
6) Addiction

Pethidine does not produce as much euphoria as morphine. Some patients show a sensitivity reaction — they feel dreadful, sweat and vomit, and have vertigo, and they may become very confused. Changing to another analgesic results in rapid improvement. Pethidine produces relaxation of smooth muscle. It may be useful for renal and biliary colic, and following large bowel surgery. It also relaxes the smooth muscle of veins — 10 mg into the drip tubing will often make the drip go if the vein is in spasm.

Pethidine is an excellent drug but may be required in greater quantities than are usually prescribed. The pain of renal colic for example may require 150—200 mg before relief is procured.

1 ml ampule containing 50 mg or 100 mg
5 ml ampule containing 50 mg (for I/V use).

Phenobarbitone

This is a long-acting barbiturate which is a sedative and tranquilliser and also has a pronounced anti-convulsant action. It is used in the treatment of eipilepsy, both prophylactically and therapeutically. Patients rapidly become tolerant to its sedative properties.

Phenoperidine (Operidine)

This is a synthetic analgesic drug derived from pethidine. It is very potent and has been developed so that it produces minimal changes in the cardiovascular system even in large doses. It has a marked respiratory depressant effect and as it acts very rapidly, it is very useful for controlling patients when they are first put on a ventilator. Its duration of action is short — approximately 2 hours when given intramuscularly, and 45 minutes when given intravenously. Phenoperidine has an emetic action and may therefore require anti-emetics to be given in combination with it. The respiratory depressant action can be reversed with nalorphine.

Phentolamine (Rogitine)

An alpha-adrenergic blocking agent which is also a direct myocardial stimulant. Adrenaline causes peripheral vasoconstriction, so blocking this effect produces vasodilatation. This will cause an increase in the *capacity* of the circulation but the *volume* circulating remains unaltered; as a result the venous return, cardiac output and arterial pressure will fall unless extra fluid is given to increase the circulating blood volume. Phentolamine is used

1) to promote vasodilatation, e.g. during cardio-pulmonary by-pass
2) to antagonise vasoconstriction, e.g. during gram negative septicaemia
3) as a direct myocardial stimulant — the vasodilatation being antagonised by Noradrenaline
4) to antagonise the vasoconstrictive effects of Noradrenaline
5) to control acute hypertensive attacks in patients with phaeochromocytoma.

1 ml ampule containing 10 mg.

Phenytoin (Epanutin, Dilantin)

This is a potent anti-convulsant agent. It tends to have less sedative action than phenobarbitone with which it is often given. It can also be used in the treatment of ventricular dysrhythmias although its action is somewhat unpredictable.

Vials containing 250 mg of powder supplied with 5 ml ampule of fluid for preparing intramuscular and intravenous injection. The solution takes some time to prepare.

Also capsules, tablets and a suspension.

Practolol (Eraldin)

Practolol is a beta-adrenergic blocking agent. Stimulation of beta receptors causes an increase in the heart rate and in myocardial contractility, and relaxation of smooth muscle. Beta blockade will therefore produce a slowing of the heart rate. Practolol is useful because it does *not* cause bronchospasm (as might be expected) so it can be used in asthmatic patients.

Ampules of 5 ml containing 10 mg (2 mg/ml)

Tablets of 100 mg.

Procaine amide

Procaineamide has a similar action to lignocaine in controlling ventricular dysrhythmias. It reduces the excitability, contractility and conductivity of the myocardium. It can be given orally and may be used to depress myocardial excitability for two weeks or so following myocardial infarction in patients who have required intravenous lignocaine to control their dysrhythmia.

Propranolol (Inderal)

Propranolol is a beta-blocking agent, like practolol. It may cause bronchoconstriction, unlike practolol, so should not be used in asthmatics. Propranolol is used

1) to control ectopic beats. It is much more effective in the control of atrial ectopics than ventricular ectopics. It is particularly useful in the treatment of dysrhythmias due to digitalis overdosage.
2) to control supraventricular tachycardia.
3) to control the tachycardia which may develop when hypotensive drugs are used.

4) to control tachycardia, or ventricular dysrhythmias due to overdosage of injected adrenaline or secretion from phaeochromocytomas.
5) to reduce myocardial oxygen consumption by reducing the heart rate. The faster the heart rate, the greater the need for oxygenated blood by the myocardium. If the myocardial circulation is impaired by atheroma, the demand can exceed the supply, resulting in angina.

1 ml ampule containing 1 mg

Also tablets of 10, 40 and 80 mg.

Pyridostigmine (Mestinon)

This is an anti-cholinesterase, similar to neostigmine but with a longer duration of action. It is used in the treatment of myasthenia gravis to provide a long term action, with neostigmine being used as a booster when extra activity is expected.

Ampules of 1 ml containing 1 mg

Tablets of 60 mg.

Salbutamol (Ventolin)

Salbutamol is an adrenergic compound developed for the treatment of bronchospasm. Like all beta adrenergic drugs it may cause tachycardia. It is usually given by inhalation as an aerosol but it may be given intravenously or orally.

Having beta-adrenergic action, Salbutamol is also used as a myocardial stimulant.

Sodium bicarbonate

Metabolic acidosis develops following more than a very brief period of cardiac arrest (30–45 secs) or as a result of poor tissue perfusion. Metabolic acidosis depresses the myocardium and successful restoration of spontaneous myocardial activity is unlikely unless the acidosis is corrected. Sodium bicarbonate is given as an 8.4% solution which contains 1 mEq per ml. The initial dose is 50–100 ml. This should ideally be administered from an 100 ml bottle, not from one of the commercially available solutions of 8.4% in 500 ml containers, as it is only too easy to administer an overdose in moments of stress.

Some Drugs Used in Intensive Care

Sodium nitroprusside

Sodium nitroprusside is a very potent, rapidly acting hypotensive agent which acts as a peripheral poison. It is used to control severe hypertension. It must be given by intravenous infusion, preferably using an infusion pump or counting chamber. As it acts in 20 seconds, the blood pressure should be recorded by direct arterial cannulation. The drug is not only fast-acting but its effect is short-lived — less than 2 minutes. It is broken down to sodium thiocyanate and sodium cyanide, both of which are poisonous, so it can only be used for relatively short periods, e.g. 3–4 days.

Streptomycin

Streptomycin is a broad spectrum bacteriocidal antibiotic. Resistant organisms are becoming much more common. The main toxic effect is damage to the auditory nerve. The drug is excreted by the kidneys so the dosage must be reduced in the presence of renal failure. Streptomycin has a slight neuromuscular blocking action, so should be used with caution in myasthenic patients, and a maximum of 4 grams used when the drug is placed in the peritoneal or thoracic cavities during surgery, since its blocking effect added to that of the muscle relaxant employed during anaesthesia may prove difficult to reverse and persist for some hours.

Strophanthin G (Ouabain)

Ouabain is a cardiac glycoside similar to digoxin but with a shorter duration of action of 2 hours. It is always given intravenously. Digitalis may not necessarily improve the state of the circulation and as the effects of ouabain become apparent very quickly and the duration of action is short, the drug can be used to assess the potential effect of cardiac glycosides.

1 ml ampule containing 0.25 mg.

Suxamethonium (Succinylcholine, Anectine)

The Suxamethonium chloride molecule is in fact two molecules of acetyl choline joined together. It acts like acetyl choline by depolarising the muscle end-plate. This depolarisation is accompanied by muscle twitching. Suxamethonium acts in about 20 seconds and paralysis lasts for 3–5

minutes. It is thus a most useful drug where quick action is required and for short procedures. The disadvantages of suxamethonium are
1) it is unstable and must be kept in a refrigerator.
2) its action cannot be reversed by any other drugs.
3) it stimulates the parasympathetic nervous system, occasionally causing bradycardia and cardiac arrest.
4) it causes a rise in serum potassium which can be fatal in patients with burns or paraplegia.
5) 1 in 3000 people cannot metabolise suxamethonium, and the paralysis may last for several hours.
6) its use is not infrequently followed by muscle pain, especially if the patient is ambulant soon after its use. However, this unpleasant side-effect can almost always be eliminated by giving not less than 20 mg gallamine, 5 mg d-tubocurarine or 1 mg pancuronium *before* the suxamethonium.

2 ml ampule containing 100 mg.

Tetracycline

Tetracycline is a broad spectrum bacteriostatic antibiotic mainly used for treating chest infections. It tends to make patients feel nauseated and anorexic, and may also cause diarrhoea due to alteration of the bowel flora. If given to children it may stain teeth yellow. It has now been replaced by oxytetracycline which does not have this disadvantage and is also cheaper.

Thiopentone (Pentothal, Intraval)

Thiopentone is a short-acting barbiturate which is used to induce anaesthesia. It has a rapid onset and its actions last for about 5 minutes, although if there is no stimulation, the patient will sleep for half an hour or more. It produces respiratory depression as well as peripheral vasodilatation and a reduction in myocardial contractility, and the drug may cause severe hypotension in the sick patient. It may also cause laryngeal spasm but this is less frequent with the $2\frac{1}{2}\%$ solution than with the 5%. Thiopentone may be given rectally in children to induce anaesthesia, and in dilute solution as an infusion to control convulsions in status epilepticus.

Ampules of 20 ml capacity containing 500 mg powder — when made up with 20 ml water for injection, the solution contains 25 mg/ml. ($2\frac{1}{2}\%$ solution).

Trimetaphan (Arfonad)

Trimetaphan is a short acting ganglion blocking agent similar in action to pentolinium. It is given by intravenous infusion since the duration of action is about 4—5 minutes. It can be given intramuscularly but the effect is less predictable; large doses cause renal damage.

Vials of 5 ml containing 250 mg (50 mg/ml).

Tubocurarine (Curare, Tubarine)

Tubocurarine, commonly called curare, is a non-depolarising muscle relaxant which acts on the motor end plate by competitive inhibition with acetyl choline. Its action is fully developed after about 3—5 minutes and the relaxation, depending on the dose, lasts for about an hour. Tubocurarine has a mild ganglion blocking effect which may produce hypotension, and if used over longer periods, paralytic ileus. Tubocurarine is a muscle relaxant only — it has no sedative properties; a patient given curare who is not anaesthetised or sedated is therefore paralysed and awake.

The action of tubocurarine is reversed by neostigmine.

Ampules of 1.5 ml containing 15 mg (10 mg/ml).

7

Intravenous Feeding

J. T. Mulvein

Introduction

Intravenous feeding is becoming much more widely used, especially in Intensive Care Units. A large number of different solutions are now available and each unit uses its own regime. This short chapter is intended to explain the basic principles governing intravenous feeding so that you will understand the rationale behind any particular scheme.

Basic Requirements

An average patient resting quietly in bed requires about 2000 calories in his diet every day. In many diseases and following surgical operations, energy demands are considerably higher and 3000 calories a day are often needed. These are the same dietary requirements as a man doing heavy manual labour; if the patient does not get these calories he is being deliberately starved.

Calories can be provided by carbohydrate, fat or protein. Carbohydrate provides 4 calories per gram. Fat is the most efficient foodstuff providing 9 calories per gram but it does require carbohydrate for its effective metabolism. Alcohol provides 7 calories per gram and this explains why alcohol is used in several solutions for intravenous feeding. Protein can provide 4 calories per gram, but protein is not primarily required in the diet as a calorie source; it is normally used for the building of body protein. The average adult requires 40 to 50 grams of protein a day. If he does not get it, he will break down his own body protein and his muscles will waste. Just as the calorie requirements increase in many diseases and postoperatively, so do the protein requirements. Ideally then, a patient requiring supplementary feeding should be given 3000 calories and 100 grams of protein every day.

Intravenous Feeding

People who are ill usually have a diminished appetite and it is unusual to see a hospital patient eating a manual labourer's diet. Indeed, a little mince with jelly and ice cream is often considered adequate. If the patient won't or can't eat, then liquid food can be given through a naso-gastric tube. This technique is very useful for feeding the unconscious patient. It relies on the alimentary tract functioning properly, but in many conditions, e.g. paralytic ileus, intestinal obstruction and malabsorption, it is impossible for enough food to be absorbed from the gut. Oral and nasogastric feeding are easy, safe and simple to manage, so it is only when they are unsuitable that intravenous feeding has to be used.

The basic substances used in intravenous feeding are carbohydrate and fat to provide calories and amino acids to provide protein. The carbohydrates used are glucose, fructose and sorbitol. Ethanol or ethyl alcohol is not strictly a carbohydrate but is also conveniently considered with this group. Glucose or dextrose as it is usually called, is used in most standard intravenous fluid regimes. These standard regimes are used chiefly to replace fluid and electrolytes, not calories. A typical regime consists of one litre of normal saline and two litres of 5% dextrose daily; this provides 400 calories. 400 calories a day is a pretty slim diet. If the patient is to be fed this way for two or three days only, there is little harm done — a little starvation doesn't harm anyone. However, the patient may already be starved or he may have to be on intravenous fluids for more than two or three days. The standard regime of normal saline and 5% dextrose would then amount to deliberate, harmful starvation.

Calorie replacement

To provide 3000 calories a day using 5% dextrose would take 15 litres of fluid. The logical answer to this problem would appear to be to use more concentrated solutions of dextrose, say 10% or 20% solutions. Concentrated *dextrose* solutions are very irritant to veins so that they thrombose rapidly; in addition these strong solutions produce glycosuria which causes an osmotic diuresis, resulting in dehydration of the patient. Finally, reactive hypoglycaemia due to insulin may occur when infusion is stopped. For these three reasons concentrated solutions of dextrose are unsuitable for use in intravenous feeding.

Fructose causes less thrombophlebitis than glucose although it is still irritant to the veins. Fructose is metabolised more rapidly in the liver than glucose so there is less urinary excretion and less diuretic effect. Fructose is also less dependant on insulin for its initial metabolism. It is usually given as a 20% or 30% solution.

Sorbitol is closely related to fructose. It is usually given as a 30% solution — a 500 ml bottle providing 600 calories. It is less irritant to the veins than fructose and has the advantage that it does not caramelise when autoclaved. The urinary losses and diuretic effect are greater than fructose but much less than glucose. Like fructose it is not dependant on insulin for its metabolism.

Ethanol (Alcohol) is useful as a calorie source, providing 7 calories per gram. Its disadvantages are that concentrations greater than 3% are irritant to veins and that if too much is given the patient may become drunk. And drunks can be uncomfortably aggressive.

Fat is very useful foodstuff for intravenous feeding as it provides the greatest number of calories in the smallest volume of fluid. Fats are insoluble in water and so must be given intravenously in the form of an emulsion. The fats commonly used are soya bean oil and cotton seed oil. Oil is not compatible with the circulation and must be first broken up into very fine droplets. This is called emulsifying and can be done physically (by shaking) or chemically (using emulsifying agents). For parenteral use, emulsifying agents are employed because the oil must *remain* as an emulsion which it will not do if merely shaken up. Egg yolk phosphatide or soya lecithin are the emulsifying agents used. The emulsion produced has to be very fine if toxic effects are to be avoided; the usual particle size is 0.7 microns. No substances should be added to fat emulsions for fear of 'cracking' the emulsion so that the solids precipitate out. Fats are more likely to cause problems with toxic effects than the other agents used in intravenous feeding. Pyrexia, chills and nausea may occur immediately on starting the drip, so when fats are given the drip should be run as slowly as possible and the patient watched closely for the first ten minutes or so. Late toxic effects include anaemia, due to depression of the bone marrow, gasto-intestinal bleeding and impaired liver function. Fats should not be given intravenously to patients with severe blood dyscrasias because of the risk of bleeding, nor to diabetics because of the danger of ketosis.

Fat emulsions must be given very slowly so that the fat particles can be cleared from the blood by the liver. A reasonable rate is 500 mls in 8 hours. Slow drips are always a problem as they tend to clot so fats are best given through a Y adaptor in the giving set in conjunction with other fluids.

Protein replacement

One would think that the easiest way of giving protein intravenously would be by giving plasma or blood. It has been shown that however much plasma is given, none of it is incorporated in the body protein. Blood and plasma are completely useless for replacing losses of tissue protein. To replace tissue protein, amino acids have to be given.

Intravenous Feeding

Amino acids occur in two forms known as optical isomers.

Greek, isos — equal or similar
isomer — substance composed of the same elements in the same proportions and with the same Molecular weights — but the components making up the molecule are arranged differently.

Light waves passed through a special prism will emerge as a pencil beam of light whose vibrations are in one plane only, and the light is now said to be *polarised*. If a beam of polarised light is passed through certain solutions, the plane of the beam will be rotated a varying degree to the right or the left.

Dextro or d-amino acids rotate the plane of polarised light to the right, *laevo or l-amino acids* to the left. The importance of the two forms is that only the l-amino acids are incorporated into tissue protein; d-amino acids are either used as a source of energy or else are excreted unchanged in the urine. Amino acid solutions are prepared either by enzymatic hydrolysis (Digestion) of naturally occurring protein or else by direct chemical synthesis. Those prepared by enzymatic hydrolysis obviously contain only l-amino acids. Synthetic amino acid solutions previously containing a mixture of d- and l-amino acids are now available with l-amino acids only. Although solutions prepared by enzymatic hydrolysis contain only l-amino acids, the hydrolysis is often incomplete and peptides may be present as well; these peptides are useless and are excreted in the urine. Amino acids solution prepared by enzymatic hydrolysis are also very acid with a pH of 4.5 to 5.5 and so are very irritant to veins. It has been shown that the effects on nitrogen balance of the synthetic l-amino acid solutions has been no better than with the protein hydrolysates. As far as adult practice is concerned, the cheaper protein hydrolysate has proved perfectly satisfactory, but the newer synthetic solutions play an important part in paediatric work.

Another important difference between the two methods of preparation is the sodium content. Solutions prepared by enzymatic hydrolysis contain a lot of sodium, often as much as normal saline; those synthesized directly contain virtually no sodium. It is important to know which type of solution is being given when electrolyte requirements are worked out. As protein is synthesized from the amino acids, potassium is incorporated in the new cells so that the patient's potassium requirements are increased. The patient receiving amino acids intravenously requires 60 to 80 milli-equivalents of potassium daily to ensure that these amino acids are synthesized into tissue protein and not merely used as a source of energy.

All amino acid solutions are hypertonic and there is therefore a loss of amino acids in the urine, so they shouldn't be given too quickly — 500 mls over 4 hours is a reasonable rate.

Vitamins are a vital constituent of any diet. The patient's reserves of fat soluble vitamins (A, D, E, & K) should last for a month. Vitamins B and C must be added to any intravenous feeding regime unless they have already been incorporated in the solutions by the manufacturers.

Complications

The biggest practical problem in intravenous feeding is thrombophlebitis. All the fluids used cause some degree of thrombophlebitis. Peripheral veins will usually only last for 24 hours before the drip stops and the patient gets a sore arm. Whenever possible intravenous feeding fluids should be given into a large vein, preferably the superior vena cava, using a long intravenous catheter.

The other less common but much more serious problem is the risk of infection. All the solutions used are excellent culture media for bacteria. Before use each bottle must be checked to ensure that there are no cracks in the glass. The solutions must be clear and there should be a vacuum present in the bottle, as shown by bubbles of air rushing into the bottle when the cap is pierced. The top of the bottle must be swabbed with spirit before inserting the giving set needle and ideally a fresh giving set should be used with each new bottle. An additional safeguard is to insert a bacterial filter where the drip set is connected to the intravenous catheter so that any bacteria which may have grown will be filtered out. A bacterial filter cannot be used with fat emulsions, however, as the fat particles will be filtered out and block the drip.

Intravenous feeding is relatively contra-indicated in cardiac and renal failure because of the danger of overloading the circulation. Fats and amino acids are contra-indicated in hepatic failure because the liver cannot metabolize the nutrients provided.

Conclusion

In summary then, intravenous feeding is required in the patient whose metabolic needs are increased because of his disease and who is unable to absorb enough food from his gastro-intestinal tract. Calories are provided by giving carbohydrate solutions and if necessary fat emulsions. Protein requirements are met by giving amino acids. Electrolytes and vitamins are also required. Remember that the patient on the standard intravenous electrolyte and dextrose regime is being deliberately starved.

8

Principles Underlying Oxygen and Carbon Dioxide Transport in the Blood

All substances whether solid, liquid or gas, are made up of molecules. The molecules are in constant random motion, and the speed at which they move is increased by a rise in temperature. In *solids* the molecules are packed so close together and move so little that the substance retains a fixed shape. In *gases* the molecules are spaced far apart and move at considerable speed. A gas will therefore tend to disperse into its surroundings unless confined within a closed vessel.

Molecular movement in *liquids* varies from one to another – in some quite fast, in others, e.g. oily ones, more slowly. Some of the molecules near the surface of the liquid tend to escape to form a *vapour*. The faster the liquid molecules are moving, the more likely are the surface molecules to escape. The concentration of the vapour above the liquid surface is related to the number of molecules forming the vapour. Heating a liquid will increase its molecular velocity and therefore the number of molecules escaping from the surface. The more molecules escaping from the liquid, the greater the number which form the vapour and the greater the concentration of the vapour. The *vapour concentration* of a liquid therefore increases with a rise in temperature. If the vapour is contained in a vessel, it will exert a *pressure* which is due to the constant bombardment of the walls of the vessel by the moving vapour molecules. A rise in temperature increases molecular velocity which increases the bombardment so that the *vapour pressure* increases also. Eventually the vapour pressure becomes the same as that of the atmosphere and bubbles are seen throughout the liquid. The temperature at which this occurs is called the boiling point. At this temperature, the vapour concentration is at its maximum and the liquid will continue to boil until it has vapourised away altogether.

The speed of molecules at room temperature varies from one liquid to another, so it is obvious that some liquids vapourise more easily than others at the same temperature. If the liquid is not in a closed container, the vapour molecules will be constantly dissipated both by air currents and their own movement and their concentration above the liquid will never reach the maximum for that particular temperature — i.e. the vapour is not a *fully saturated* vapour. In the lungs water vapour is always fully saturated at the body temperature of 37°C. Since the vapour pressure of the environment is nearly always lower than that of the air in the lungs the body tends to lose water to the environment through the lungs.

Gases in solution

Just as liquid molecules can escape from the surface of a liquid to form a vapour above it, so can molecules of a gas pass into a liquid to mix or 'dissolve' in it. The number of gas molecules which pass into the liquid is related to the temperature and therefore the pressure of the gas, as well as the temperature of the liquid. The higher the gas pressure, the greater is the number of gas molecules which tend to pass into the liquid. On the other hand, the higher the temperature of the liquid, the less easy is it for the gas molecules to remain within it since they will tend to escape from the liquid, or vapourise out of it. The solubility of a *gas at room temperature* is therefore decreased in a hot liquid and increased in a cold liquid.

The gas molecules in a liquid exert a pressure in the liquid which is related to the number of molecules present and the speed at which they move about colliding with the liquid molecules and bombarding the walls of the container. This pressure is called the *gas tension* in the particular liquid. The term pressure should, strictly speaking, be used for the gaseous state.

Mixtures of gases

In a mixture of gases, each gas exerts its own pressure proportional to its concentration in the mixture and this pressure is called the Partial Pressure of that gas. The pressure of the *mixture* is the sum of all the partial pressures,

> e.g. The atmosphere or air consists mainly of Oxygen, Nitrogen and Water vapour.

Each of these gases exerts its own partial pressure and these all add up to the pressure exerted by the atmosphere. Knowing the atmospheric pressure and the concentration of the various components, it is simple to calculate their respective partial pressures. These are denoted by a capital P with the molecular symbol of the gas following, e.g. PO_2 represents the Partial pressure of Oxygen.

The pressure of the atmosphere is around 760 mmHg at sea level. As we know well, it does vary from day to day. The proportion of water vapour present also varies, as does the water vapour pressure. For accurate measurement of the partial pressure of Oxygen in air, the atmospheric pressure and the water vapour pressure at the time must be found and the water vapour pressure subtracted from the atmospheric pressure. This then gives the total pressure exerted by the *dry* gases of the atmospheric air whose proportions do not change. The PO_2 may then be calculated as follows:

The barometer reading is found to be	760 mmHg
The vapour pressure of water at a room temperature of 20°C at the time is found to be	20 mmHg
The percentage of Oxygen in air is	20%

The partial pressure of oxygen in the air is 20% of 760 − 38

$$= 20\% \text{ of } 722$$

$$= \frac{20}{100} \times 722$$

$$= 144.4 \text{ mmHg}$$

A sample of air from the alveoli contains only 14% oxygen.

Under the same barometric conditions as before, and knowing that the saturated water vapour pressure at the body temperature of 37°C is 47 mmHg,

The partial pressure of oxygen in the alveoli is 14% of 760 − 47

$$= \frac{14}{100} \times 713$$

$$= 99.8 \text{ mmHg}$$

In the alveoli, gaseous oxygen comes into very close contact with the blood. The partial pressure of oxygen in the alveoli − the alveolar PO_2 − is important because it influences the oxygenation of the blood. The tension of a gas in a liquid is directly related to the partial pressure of the gas. The higher the gas pressure, the higher the gas tension in the liquid. In the body, the arterial oxygen tension affects the relationship between oxygen and Haemoglobin which will be described.

At *sea level,* assuming an atmospheric pressure of 760 mm Hg, the alveolar PO_2 is 99.8 mmHg. At a height of *12,000 feet* above sea level, the barometric pressure is only 483 mmHg. Although the composition of the air does not change, a reduction in the atmospheric pressure means that the partial pressures of the gases of the air will all be reduced accordingly. The partial pressure of oxygen in the air will be only about 100 mmHg and the *alveolar* PO_2 reduced to about 61 mmHg. This pressure is insufficient to provide an adequate arterial oxygen tension for the efficient uptake of oxygen by the blood, although some compensation can occur, notably in the form of an increased number of red blood cells.

Oxygen carriage in the blood

Oxygen molecules 'dissolve' in the blood in the way previously described and exert a pressure proportional to the number of molecules present. The capital letter P is used to denote the partial pressure of a gas as well as its tension in a liquid. When writing, a capital letter A denotes *alveolar* pressure and a small letter a the *arterial* gas tension.

Thus PAO_2 refers to the partial pressure of oxygen in the alveoli

PaO_2 refers to the oxygen tension of arterial blood.

The amount of oxygen present as free molecules 'dissolved' in the blood is approximately 0.3 ml per 100 ml of blood. Such a quantity is quite inadequate to provide for the metabolic needs of the body. A far greater quantity of oxygen is able to be absorbed by the blood as a result of a chemical combination between oxygen and Haemoglobin.

Every molecule of Haemoglobin (Hb) is able to take up 4 molecules of oxygen. If 4 molecules of oxygen combine with 1 molecule of Hb, the Hb is *fully saturated.*

Every *gram* of Hb when fully saturated carries 1.3 ml oxygen. If the average fit person contains 15 grams of Hb per 100 ml of blood, and that Hb is fully saturated with oxygen, 100 ml of arterial blood will contain $15 \times 1.3 = 19.5$ ml oxygen.

The extent to which Hb is saturated — the percentage saturation — depends on the pulmonary arterial oxygen tension. If the arterial oxygen tension is the normal of 95—98 mmHg, then the Hb is nearly fully saturated at 95—97%. If the arterial oxygen tension is reduced, so is the Hb saturation — but it is reduced in a peculiar way. By taking samples of blood and exposing them to oxygen at different pressures, a graph may be constructed which shows the relationship between the partial pressure of oxygen and the extent to which the Hb molecules are saturated with oxygen. The S-shaped curve of this graph is known as the Oxygen Dissociation curve.

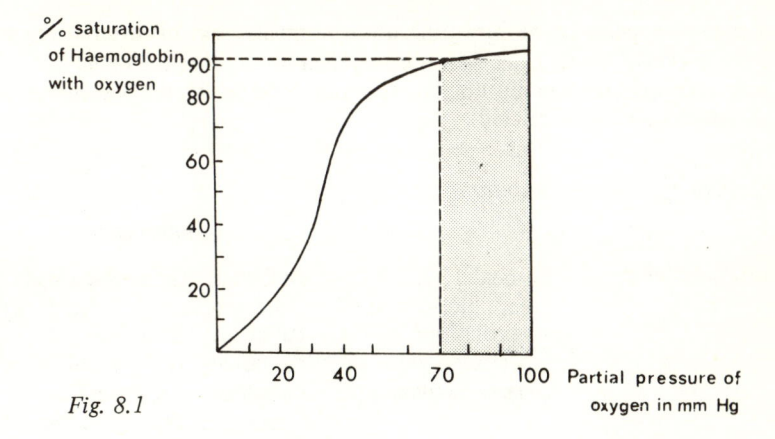

Principles Underlying Oxygen and Carbon Dioxide Transport

Fig. 8.1

The top 'flat' portion shows that a reduction of the partial pressure of oxygen down to 70 mmHg produces very little change in the saturation of Hb. At a PO_2 of 70 mmHg the saturation is still about 90%. In other words, the oxygen tension in the pulmonary capillaries can drop to 70 mmHg before the uptake of oxygen by Hb begins to be affected to any great extent.

Arterial oxygen saturation

The blood in the pulmonary veins *leaving* the lungs is not more than 93–95% saturated. This is due to the fact that the *ventilation* of the alveoli and the *perfusion* of the pulmonary capillaries is not uniform, even in normal lungs. Local variations in the ratio between ventilation and perfusion occur as a result of sleep, activity and changes in posture. The ventilation/perfusion ratio becomes more irregular in disease. Furthermore, some blood never goes through the lungs (veins in the myocardial walls draining directly into the ventricles, and some of the bronchial veins which drain via the pulmonary veins into the left atrium). All these factors create a 'shunt' of up to 5% — that is, 5% of the blood in the left side of the heart will be venous blood, and will, by mixing with the oxygenated blood from the lungs, reduce the overall saturation of systemic arterial blood.

Venous admixture

This term is used to account for the difference between the oxygen tension in the pulmonary end-capillary blood and the systemic arterial blood. The term venous admixture is really a tidy medical concept. If a patient appears to be breathing quite normally, but his arterial oxygen tension (PaO_2) is reduced below normal, then we say that the reduction in oxygen tension must be due to venous admixture, the percentage of which can be calculated.

Sources of venous admixture

	Normal	Abnormal
Intrapulmonary	Bronchial veins Fluctuations in the ventilation/perfusion ratio in sleep, activity etc.	Atalectasis (scattered small areas of unventilated lung) Pulmonary infection Pulmonary A–V shunt Pulmonary neoplasm Circulation through damaged, contused or oedematous lung.
Extra-pulmonary	Veins in the myocardium	Congenital heart disease associated with right to left shunting.

The release of oxygen into the tissues

At an arterial oxygen tension of 40 mmHg the Hb saturation is still over 70%. A reduction of only 10 mmHg in the arterial tension – from

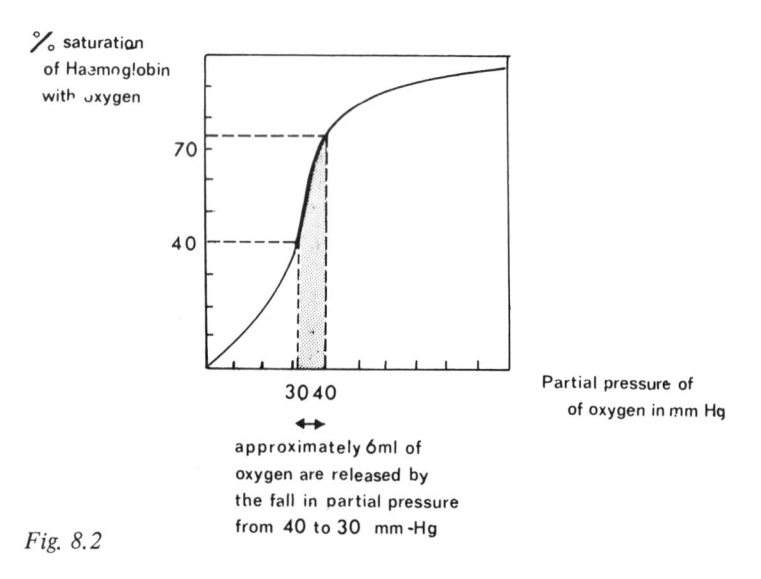

Fig. 8.2

approximately 6ml of oxygen are released by the fall in partial pressure from 40 to 30 mm-Hg

Principles Underlying Oxygen and Carbon Dioxide Transport 101

40 to 30 — causes the Hb saturation to fall from 74% to 40%. This large change in saturation in response to a small change in tension causes the release of *over a quarter* of the oxygen molecules carried by the Hb.

Since the oxygen tension of the interstitial fluid bathing the tissues is about 35 mmHg at rest and drops almost to zero in extreme exertion, the rapid dissociation of Hb when the blood reaches the tissues is excellently suited to the metabolic needs of the body.

You will remember that matter is made up of atoms of *elements*, e.g. Hydrogen, Carbon, Sodium, Oxygen.

Atoms are composed of a central positively-charged nucleus surrounded by a number of negatively-charged *electrons*. The nucleus is made up of *protons* and *neutrons*. The positive charge on the nucleus is due to the presence of the protons. Neutrons, as their name implies, are electrically neutral. The number of electrons is equal to the number of protons, so that the total atom is electrically neutral. Variation in the number of neutrons in the nucleus produces *isotopes*.

If an atom loses an electron, it becomes positively charged. If an electron is gained, the atom becomes negatively charged. Atoms carrying an electrical charge are called *ions*.

Substances are composed of *molecules*. The Hydrogen molecule consists of two atoms of hydrogen, and a molecule of Carbon Dioxide consists of one atom of carbon and two atoms of oxygen. Some of the common elements, molecules and ions with their symbols which are met in physiology are shown below.

Elements		*Molecules*		*Ions*	
Hydrogen	H	Hydrogen	H_2	Hydrogen	H^+
Oxygen	O	Oxygen	O_2	Sodium	Na^+
Sodium	Na (Natrium)	Nitrogen	N_2	Potassium	K^+
Carbon	C	Carbon dioxide	CO_2	Chloride	Cl'
Potassium	K (Kalium)	Sodium Chloride	NaCl	Bicarbonate	HCO_3'
Iron	Fe (Ferrum)	Water	H_2O		
Calcium	Ca				
Nitrogen	N				
Chlorine	Cl				

Electrolytes are substances such as sodium chloride which exist as sodium and chloride ions rather than as a molecule, even in the solid state. According to Brønsted, substances which produce Hydrogen ions H^+ are called acids. Those substances which will accept or take up H^+ are called bases. Modern theories are more complex, but the principle is essentially similar and is useful in explaining the transport of carbon dioxide in the blood.

Carbon dioxide CO_2 can react with water to form carbonic acid H_2CO_3 which then dissociates into hydrogen ions H^+ and bicarbonate ions HCO_3'.

$$CO_2 + H_2O \rightarrow H_2CO_3 \rightarrow H^+ + HCO_3'$$

Excessive variation in the hydrogen ion concentration in the cells and body fluids, particularly in the blood, is incompatible with human life. The elimination of excess hydrogen ions from the body and the maintainance of the normal range of concentration is therefore of great importance. The body can *excrete* hydrogen ions only through the kidney. The ability to do this is restricted, and hydrogen ions while waiting to be excreted must be neutralised electrically. This process is called *buffering*. The hydrogen ions associated with the transport of carbon dioxide from the tissues to the lungs do not however be required to be excreted as hydrogen ions. They need only to be buffered efficiently until they reform carbon dioxide and water in the lungs.

Carbon dioxide is present in the blood in various forms.

1) In physical 'solution' as free molecules. These molecules are responsible for exerting the carbon dioxide tension of the blood.
2) As carbonic acid (H_2CO_3) in small quantities in the plasma.
3) As carbamino compounds both in the plasma and in the red cells. Amino groups (a combination of Nitrogen and Hydrogen) can combine directly with carbon dioxide. The protein Haemoglobin combines with quite a lot of carbon dioxide in this way.
4) As *bicarbonate ion* HCO_3'.

Most of the carbon dioxide molecules produced as a result of metabolic activity are carried in this form. Carbon dioxide molecules are able to pass across cell membranes very rapidly and have no difficulty in diffusing from tissue cells, through the interstitial fluid into the blood, and into the red blood cells.

Inside the red cells, the reaction between carbon dioxide and water, normally a very slow one, is enormously speeded up under the influence of the enzyme carbonic anhydrase. The carbonic acid formed dissociates immediately to form hydrogen ions and bicarbonate ions.

$$CO_2 + H_2O \rightarrow H_2CO_3 \rightarrow H^+ + HCO_3'.$$

The build-up of bicarbonate ions inside the cell creates a *concentration gradient* across the cell membrane, i.e. there are more bicarbonate ions on one side of the cell membrane than the other. As a result, the bicarbonate ions diffuse out across the cell membrane into the plasma. The cell membrane however is less permeable to the passage of hydrogen ions so that their concentration rises within the cells. Since the bicarbonate ions are passing out of the cells under the influence of the concentration gradient, their disappearance creates an excess of positively-charged ions (H^+) within the cells. The majority of these hydrogen ions are accepted by Haemoglobin molecules, and in order to restore and maintain an *electrical* equilibrium, chloride ions Cl' from the plasma pass into the red cells in exchange for the bicarbonate ions HCO_3'.

In this way, the carbon dioxide molecules are transported in the blood to the lungs. There, the carbon dioxide tension in the blood entering the pulmonary capillaries is higher than that in the alveoli. Carbon dioxide molecules in 'solution' therefore diffuse out of the blood into the alveoli and in so doing stimulate the reversal of the process just described. Bicarbonate ions pass back into the red cells, join with hydrogen ions to form carbonic acid which then splits up to form carbon dioxide and water. The carbon dioxide molecules diffuse out into the alveoli to be breathed out into the atmosphere and the chloride ions pass back into the plasma.

Arterial Blood gas measurement

Arterial blood samples are taken from an indwelling arterial cannula if present, or by percutaneous arterial puncture. The radial and femoral arteries are usually employed although some prefer the brachial. A 5 ml syringe, a syringe cap, No. 1 needle, and heparin 1000 units/ml are required together with spirit and some swabs. Only enough heparin is required to fill the 'dead space' of the syringe and needle.

Immediately after sampling, the syringe is sealed with the cap in order to exclude air as the blood gas tensions will gradually alter if the syringe is left unsealed. The syringe should be immersed in *iced-water* in a thermos flask pending analysis which should be performed as soon as possible to ensure accurate results. Never leave the syringe in the ward fridge — the interior is not cold enough (commonly about 48—54°F) and in any case the sample is bound to be forgotten. Temporary storage in the ice-box will not lower the temperature of the sample quickly enough and if the sample is forgotten, the blood will then be frozen solid. On the whole, arterial blood is analysed in order to check on the adequacy of ventilation or oxygenation. In principle therefore, samples should not be taken unless analysis will be performed promptly so that alterations, if necessary, may be made in

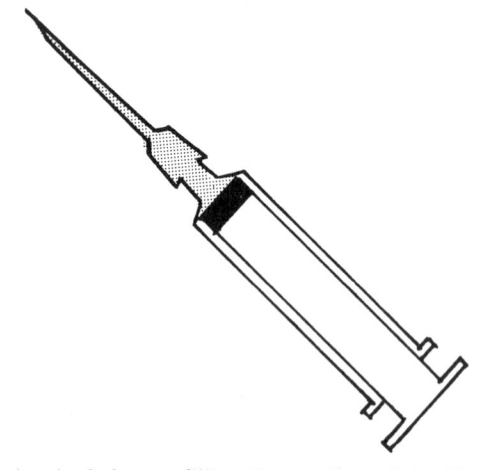

Fig. 8.3 Heparin, shaded grey, filling the needle and the 'dead space' of the syringe.

the patient's treatment as soon as possible. Any prolonged delay between sampling and analysis implies that the investigation is unnecessary.

Following arterial puncture, firm pressure must be exerted over the puncture area for at least 5 minutes in order to avoid unnecessary haemorrhage. It is possible for several punctures to be made in the radial artery without causing residual swelling or bruising provided that application of pressure is conscientiously observed. This is particularly important when repeated arterial puncture is required, since swelling around the artery makes localisation and successful puncture more difficult, and an alternative site might have to be used sooner than necessary.

If an arterial cannula is present, then 3 syringes are required; one to 'clear' the cannula of heparinised saline prior to taking the arterial sample in the 2nd heparinised syringe, and the 3rd to flush the cannula with heparinised saline afterwards.

Results of analysis

pH value   This is a term used to express the acidity or alkalinity of solutions and is related to the hydrogen ion concentration of the solution. As the hydrogen ion concentration of a solution increases, so does its acidity. The pH range however works in reverse because of the way the pH value is calculated.

Type of solution	Acid	Alkaline
pH value	1 2 3 4 5 6	7 8 9 10 11
Hydrogen ion concentration	High	Low

Thus a solution with a pH value of 7.30 is more acid than one with a value of 7.56. The normal range of pH value for arterial blood is 7.36 to 7.44. If the blood pH is less than 7.34, the patient is said to be acidotic; when the pH value is greater than 7.44, the patient is alkalotic.

Owing to the fact that carbon dioxide stimulates the formation of hydrogen ions, a low pH value – acidosis – can be due to an excess of carbon dioxide in the blood associated with underventilation. On the other hand it may be due to the presence of excess acid metabolites, metabolic disease or renal failure. The pH value alone cannot therefore differentiate between respiratory and metabolic acidosis.

PaCO$_2$ The carbon dioxide tension in arterial blood, commonly abbreviated to PCO$_2$. The normal range for arterial blood is 36–44 mmHg. When the PCO$_2$ is greater than 44 mmHg, it indicates that the patient is unable to eliminate carbon dioxide satisfactorily. The patient, by definition, is in respiratory failure. The excess carbon dioxide leads to an increase in the hydrogen ion concentration of the blood so that the pH value falls, and the patient is said to have a respiratory acidosis. Respiratory failure can be acute or chronic. Acute respiratory failure, unrelieved spontaneously or by treatment, results in death. Chronic respiratory failure may be seen in the elderly bronchitic who manages to compensate physiologically for his diseased lungs. The kidney increases its excretion of hydrogen ions and *retains* HCO$_3'$ since they can help to 'buffer' the excessive number of hydrogen ions produced by the excess carbon dioxide. The chronic bronchitic will therefore have a raised PCO$_2$ (in the 50–60 mmHg range), an increased plasma bicarbonate level and a pH near normal.

Standard Bicarbonate

This is the concentration of bicarbonate ions in the arterial blood, measured in mEq/l (milliequivalents per litre), at a PCO$_2$ of 40 mmHg and a temperature of 37°C. The normal range is 22–26 mEq/l.

When the patient's PCO_2 is outside the normal limit, the bicarbonate levels will vary according to the actual PCO_2 and the patient's ability to cope with the situation. A special chart is used to tell us what the bicarbonate level *would* be at the standard PCO_2 of 40 mmHg.

Base excess or base deficit — normal range +2.5 to −2.5 mEq/l

This gives an indication of the metabolic state of the patient, i.e. whether he is acidotic or alkalotic from the metabolic aspect. As we have seen, carbon dioxide acts as an acid in the body, and the pH of the blood will reflect variations from the normal both from respiratory abnormalities as well as tissue metabolism. Base excess or deficit refers to tissue metabolism only.

Haemoglobin saturation   Normal range 95–98%

PaO_2 The oxygen tension of arterial blood   Normal range 80–104 mmHg.

9

The Regulation of Hydrogen Ion Concentration and Acid-Base Balance

This is a difficult subject to grasp and describe because the cells and fluids of the body constitute a complex metabolic system. So many activities go on at the same time that it does not make it easy to discuss any one particular aspect.

The many substances making up the body range from complex protein molecules to ions such as sodium, chloride and hydrogen, and the metabolic activities result in a constant biochemical turnover. Substances taken in as food are broken down to an acceptable biochemical state, any constituents required are absorbed and assimilated, and those in excess or unwanted are excreted. The metabolic processes of the body are such that there is a tendency for it to become acid; at the same time, the amount or concentration of many of the biochemical constituents must be maintained within fairly narrow limits in spite of constant metabolic activity. Variations in *acid-base balance*, whether normal or pathological, are probably more easily understood if they are considered primarily in terms of *hydrogen ion* concentration; but it is important to realise that change in the concentrations of *other* ions will also affect hydrogen ion concentration and conversely, variation in hydrogen ion concentration will induce changes in other ions.

ACIDS are substances which produce hydrogen ions; bases are substances which will accept hydrogen ions. Confusion will arise if this definition is not kept absolutely clear. The reason is simple; physiologists, chemists and clinicians used different terminology for many years and even today, some people still tend to think of negative ions as 'acidic' and positive ions as 'basic'. The following examples should show how such an approach will cause confusion:

Hydrochloric acid — symbol HCl — is an electrically neutral substance which is dissociated completely into an equal number of hydrogen ions and chloride ions.

$$HCl \rightarrow H^+ + Cl'$$

The di-hydrogen phosphate ion — H_2PO_4'' — is a negative ion or anion. It can dissociate into a hydrogen ion and a mono-hydrogen phosphate ion. When it does so, it is acting as an acid.

$$H_2PO_4'' \rightarrow H^+ + HPO_4'$$

di-hydrogen phosphate ion   mono-hydrogen phosphate ion

The ammonium ion — NH_4^+ — is a positive ion or cation. It can dissociate into a hydrogen ion and a molecule of ammonia.

$$NH_4^+ \rightarrow H^+ + NH_3$$

These three examples show that an acid can be an electrically neutral substance, a negative ion, or a positive ion. The thing they have in common is that they can produce hydrogen ions. Ions such as sodium or potassium are neither acids nor bases since they cannot produce or accept hydrogen ions.

The other basic rule is that the body always strives to maintain an electrical balance, neutrality, or equilibrium, amongst the many ions present — in other words, the total number of positive ions are matched by negative ions, although the numbers of individual ions varies considerably. If extra hydrogen ions are produced as a result of metabolic processes, they must be neutralised by negative ions, assimilated into other ions or formed into neutral molecules until they can be excreted by the kidney.

Some acids — strong acids — dissociate completely into their constituent ionic radicals; others are only partly dissociated, and a solution of such an acid, e.g. carbonic acid H_2CO_3 will contain undissociated carbonic acid molecules as well as hydrogen and bicarbonate ions.

$$H_2CO_3 \rightleftharpoons H^+ + HCO_3'$$

The extent of dissociation varies with the chemical environment and the double arrow indicates that the chemical reaction can, and does, proceed in either direction and that at any one time both the molecule and its ions are present. An increase in concentration of any one of the participants of the reaction will tend to induce further dissociation or a

Regulation of Hydrogen Ion Concentration and Acid-Base Balance

reduction in the number of dissociated ions accordingly,

> An increase in the amount of carbonic acid will lead to an increase in dissociation and the production of hydrogen ions
>
> $$H_2CO_3 \rightleftharpoons H^+ + HCO_3'$$

e.g. increasing the number of hydrogen ions present will tend to promote the formation of carbonic acid molecules

$$H_2CO_3 \rightleftharpoons H^+ + HCO_3'$$

Acids whose dissociation is incomplete are known as weak acids. The fact that the dissociation varies according to the concentration of their constituent particles means that they can respond to a *change* in their chemical environment if the change involves one of their constituents — in other words, they can act as *buffers* to resist a change in the ionic concentration of their environment. A buffer is a system of an acid and a base in which the acid is incompletely dissociated,

$$\text{e.g. } H_2CO_3 \rightleftharpoons H^+ + HCO_3'$$
$$\quad\quad\quad \text{acid} \quad\quad\quad \text{base}$$

Three mechanisms are available to the body to help it maintain the normal physiological range of hydrogen ion concentration.

1) Buffer systems
2) Excretion of hydrogen ions via the kidney
3) The regulation of carbon dioxide excretion through the lungs. Although carbon dioxide is not an acid by definition, i.e. it itself is not a hydrogen ion donor, it acts as a source of hydrogen ions due to the mechanisms by which it is removed from the body — and these mechanisms can also act as a buffer system in the extracellular fluid to control variations in hydrogen ion concentration produced by other metabolic processes.

Carbon dioxide excretion

Carbon dioxide and water are the end products of many metabolic processes. The carbon dioxide is ultimately excreted in the lungs but is mainly transported there from the tissues in the form of bicarbonate ions,

$$H_2O + CO_2 \rightleftharpoons H_2CO_3 \rightleftharpoons H^+ + HCO_3'$$

In the lung capillaries, the chemical reaction tends to proceed in the reverse direction so that carbon dioxide is reformed,

$$H^+ + HCO_3' \rightleftharpoons H_2CO_3 \rightleftharpoons H_2O + CO_2$$
$$\text{excreted by the kidney} \quad\quad\quad \text{excreted by the lungs}$$

The reactions take place *in the red cells* and as the concentration of hydrogen and bicarbonate ions builds up within the cells in the tissue capillaries, the bicarbonate ions pass out into the plasma, leaving the hydrogen ions within the cells. These 'free' hydrogen ions are buffered by Haemoglobin molecules whose ability to do so is related to whether or not the Haemoglobin is oxygenated. Oxygenated Haemoglobin is a weak base, whereas reduced Haemoglobin (Haemoglobin without its oxygen) is a strong base and readily accepts hydrogen ions. The removal of oxygen from Haemoglobin in the tissue capillaries simultaneously provides an effective buffer for the hydrogen ions of carbonic acid Haemoglobin thus plays a very important part in the transport of carbon dioxide from the tissues to the lungs. The reaction

$$H_2O + CO_2 \rightarrow H_2CO_3 \rightarrow H^+ + HCO_3'$$

cannot proceed fully to the right unless the hydrogen ions are removed as well as the bicarbonate ions. The removal of hydrogen ions by reduced Haemoglobin encourages the reaction to proceed as far as is necessary to remove the carbon dioxide from the tissues, and at the same time minimises the rise in hydrogen ion concentration in the blood which would otherwise occur.

In the lungs, the whole process is reversed; the re-formed carbon dioxide is excreted and the hydrogen ions 'disappear'. Disappear electrically, that is. They are present all the time, actually or potentially, in the molecules of water and carbonic acid and are only revealed when the bicarbonate ions are removed from the environment. Remember that hydrogen ions cannot be removed from the body via the lungs — they can only be excreted by the kidney.

Buffers

As carbonic acid is the acid formed in the largest quantity in the body, the importance of Haemoglobin as an intracellular buffer is obvious. Haemoglobin can, of course, buffer acids produced by other metabolic processes, as can the plasma proteins, although their capacity for buffering is much less.

In the extra cellular fluid compartment, the carbonic acid/bicarbonate system is available to resist changes in H^+ ion concentration, i.e. to act as a buffer.

$$H^+ + HCO_3' \rightleftharpoons H_2CO_3 \rightleftharpoons H_2O + CO_2$$
excreted by the kidney   excreted by the lungs

An increase in hydrogen ion concentration will cause the reaction to proceed to the right, and a decrease in hydrogen ion concentration will cause the reaction to proceed to the left. It is important to realise that this reaction takes place in the interstitial fluid and the

Regulation of Hydrogen Ion Concentration and Acid-Base Balance 111

Disturbances of acid-base balance

Acidosis	Respiratory Metabolic
Alkalosis	Respiratory Metabolic

Some of the symbols used in association with these disturbances;

- $P_A CO_2$ — the partial pressure of carbon dioxide in the blood
- $P_a CO_2$ — the carbon dioxide tension in the arterial blood
- PCO_2 — may refer to either or both the above
- pH — a measure of hydrogen ion concentration.

plasma, as well as the red cells. The molecules of carbonic acid are in equilibrium with molecules of carbon dioxide dissolved in the plasma, and it is this particular chemical equilibrium which makes the carbonic acid/bicarbonate buffer system so effective. The partial pressure of carbon dioxide in the alveoli determines the carbon dioxide gas tension in the pulmonary arterial blood. The word tension is employed when a gas exerts a pressure in a liquid, i.e. when it is dissolved. Hence, a rise in carbon dioxide tension in the blood arriving in the lungs, due to an increase in the number of dissolved carbon dioxide molecules following a rise in extracellular H^+ ion concentration, will produce a rise in alveolar carbon dioxide pressure; this will stimulate an increase in pulmonary ventilation and the removal of the excess carbon dioxide. The excess hydrogen ions are excreted by the kidney, but this is a slower process and the buffering action of the carbonic acid/bicarbonate system helps to maintain a normal range of hydrogen ion concentration while renal excretion takes place.

Respiratory acidosis

This condition is synonymous with ventilatory failure. Inadequate ventilation of the lungs means that the carbon dioxide reformed as a result of the reaction

$$H^+ + HCO_3' \rightleftharpoons H_2CO_3 \rightleftharpoons H_2O + CO_2$$

fails to be removed, so the alveolar and arterial PCO_2 rise. The equilibrium of the reaction is altered, causing it to proceed to the left, so there is an increase in the concentration of carbonic acid, and a rise in hydrogen ion concentration, in the blood. These hydrogen ions will be buffered by plasma bicarbonate ions, but many more are needed than are available, and the kidney responds by retaining bicarbonate ions and excreting hydrogen ions to the best of its ability. The actual rise in blood hydrogen ion concentration will depend on the rapidity and severity of the ventilatory failure. In chronic respiratory disease, compensation by the kidney is often adequate to maintain the blood hydrogen ion concentration within normal limits; in acute respiratory failure, the effects of carbon dioxide retention are so great that the kidney cannot compensate effectively — the rate of accumulation of hydrogen ions is far greater than the rate at which the kidney can excrete them.

Blood gas analysis will show — a rise in hydrogen ion concentration
i.e. a fall in pH value
concentration if compensation occurs, i.e. there is a *compensatory metabolic alkalosis.*

Metabolic acidosis
This will follow
1) an increase in acid in the extracellular fluid
2) a loss of base from the extracellular fluid.

Acids in the extracellular fluid may be increased by dietary intake, metabolic processes or failure of renal excretion. The condition does *not* include an increase in *carbonic* acid resulting from increased tissue production of carbon dioxide.

Significant loss of the alkaline alimentary secretions through diarrhoea or a biliary fistula will reduce the concentration of *bases* in the extracellular fluid.

An increase in hydrogen ions in the extracellular fluid is buffered by the bicarbonate ions which leads to the formation of carbonic acid and a fall in bicarbonate ion concentration.

$$H^+ + HCO_3' \rightarrow H_2CO_3$$

This might be expected to produce an increase in plasma carbonic acid concentration and therefore in the arterial and alveolar PCO_2

$$H_2CO_3 \rightarrow CO_2 + H_2O \text{ but this is not seen because}$$

1) the excess carbon dioxide produced from the carbonic acid is easily removed by the lungs
2) the raised hydrogen ion concentration stimulates such an increase in pulmonary ventilation that the alveolar and arterial PCO_2, and therefore the carbonic acid concentration, are actually reduced.

The response to a metabolic acidosis is thus a *respiratory alkalosis* — i.e. a reduced PCO_2. The induced fall in PCO_2 actually augments the buffering activity of bicarbonate ions, since reducing the concentration of dissolved carbon dioxide in the blood (the arterial PCO_2) encourages the reaction to proceed more fully to the right;

$$H^+ + HCO_3' \rightarrow H_2CO_3 \rightarrow H_2O + CO_2 \text{ excreted in the lungs}$$

Buffering of hydrogen ions by bicarbonate ions, augmented by the respiratory response to the rise in hydrogen ion concentration, will compensate for minor degrees of metabolic acidosis until the kidney is able to excrete the excess hydrogen ions. Where compensation has occurred, blood gas analysis will reveal a low PCO_2, a low bicarbonate ion concentration and a hydrogen ion concentration within normal limits.

Respiratory alkalosis

This is due to excessive pulmonary ventilation which lowers the PCO_2 below the normal range. Some of the causes are

voluntary or artificial hyperventilation
pathological hyperventilation due to anoxia, cerebral disease, salicylate poisoning, diabetic ketosis etc.

Hyperventilation leads to a fall in PCO_2 which induces a fall in both hydrogen and bicarbonate ion concentration in the blood.

$$H^+ + HCO_3' \rightarrow H_2CO_3 \rightarrow H_2O + CO_2 \text{ excreted in the lungs}$$

Hydrogen ion concentration must be maintained within normal limits so the kidney responds by reabsorbing more hydrogen ions. This is a relatively slow process, but a further increase in hydrogen ion concentration is obtained by renal secretion of bicarbonate ions, reducing still further the concentration of bicarbonate ions in the plasma. The response to a respiratory alkalosis is therefore a metabolic acidosis (due here to a reduction in base) augmenting the fall in bicarbonate ion concentration initially caused by the fall in PCO_2. Whether or not an alkalaemia occurs will depend on the rapidity of development of the respiratory alkalosis — if it is acute, the kidney cannot respond quickly enough and the blood hydrogen ion concentration remains low — alkalaemia. In the chronic state, compensation by the kidney will usually maintain the blood pH within the normal range although at the alkaline end of it.

Metabolic alkalosis

This follows a decrease in the concentration of acids *other than carbonic acid* in the extracellular fluid, or an increase of base.

Loss of acid occurs in vomiting, or in conditions of potassium depletion when the kidney excretes hydrogen ions in order to retain potassium ions instead.

Increase in base will follow excessive administration of sodium bicarbonate and similar substances.

Loss of acid causes a fall in hydrogen ion concentration and tends to induce the reaction

$$H^+ + HCO_3' \rightleftharpoons H_2CO_3 \rightleftharpoons H_2O + CO_2$$

to proceed to the left.

This would reduce the PCO_2, but in fact, it usually remains within normal limits because the reduced hydrogen ion concentration depresses pulmonary ventilation. The slight shift of equilibrium to the left helps to raise the hydrogen ion concentration towards normal. Bicarbonate ion concentration is of course increased at the same time.

An increase in base would be expected to cause the reaction to proceed to the right

$$H^+ + HCO_3' \rightarrow H_2CO_3 \rightarrow H_2O + CO_2$$

producing a rise in PCO_2 but this seldom happens.

In metabolic alkalosis, alkalaemia (a reduced hydrogen ion concentration in the blood) is nearly always present, together with an increased concentration of bicarbonate ion in the plasma.

10

Physical Chemistry, Osmotic Pressure and Osmolarity

Matter is made up of basic *elements*, e.g. Hydrogen, Sodium, Oxygen, Carbon. *Atoms* of elements are composed of a central, positively-charged nucleus surrounded by a number of negatively-charged *electrons*.

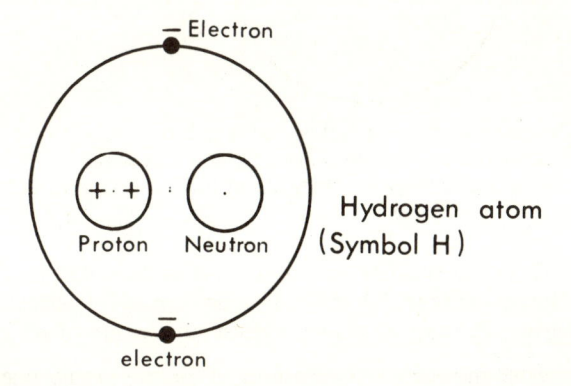

Fig. 10.1 Hydrogen atom (Symbol H)

The nucleus itself is made up of *protons* and *neutrons*. The mass or weight of the nucleus is due to the presence of both protons and neutrons — but the positive charge on the nucleus is due to the presence of the protons only. Neutrons, as the name implies, are electrically neutral. The negative charge of the electrons is exactly equal to the positive charge of the nucleus so that the total atom is electrically neutral.

The number of protons in the nucleus of an atom of an element is equal to the number of surrounding electrons, and this number, the *atomic number*, is responsible for the *chemical* behaviour of the element

116 *Intensive Care for Nurses*

concerned. Every atom of every element has the same number of protons and electrons — but the number of neutrons in the nucleus of the particular atom can vary. Since the *weight* of an atom is due mainly to the protons and neutrons (the weight of the electrons is negligible by comparison) it is possible for the *atomic weight* of an element to vary, although its *atomic number* does not. The variations in the number of neutrons in the nucleus, and therefore in the atomic weight, produces *isotopes* of an element.

If an atom loses an electron it becomes positively charged. If an electron is gained, the atom becomes negatively charged. Atoms carrying an electrical charge are called *ions*.

Hydrogen ion (Symbol H^+)

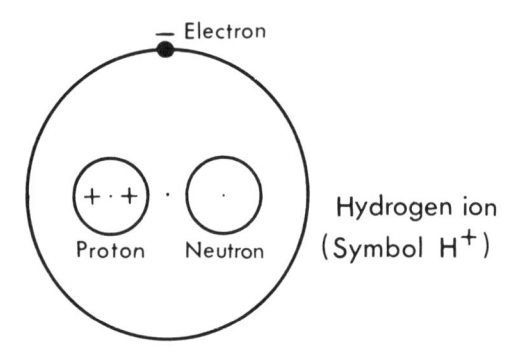

Fig. 10.2 The loss of one negatively-charged electron means that the incomplete atom — now called an ion — has two positive charges and only one negative charge, and the ion is now therefore positively charged.

A *molecule* is the smallest particle of a substance that is capable of a separate stable existence. A molecule may consist of one atom only, e.g. the element Helium; or it may consist of a group of different atoms,

e.g. the water molecule — two atoms of Hydrogen and one atom of Oxygen

the sodium bicarbonate molecule — one atom each of Sodium, Hydrogen and Carbon, and three atoms of Oxygen.

Note that the term molecule may refer either to an element or a compound of atoms — it is correct to speak of a molecule of Oxygen (consisting of two atoms of Oxygen) or a molecule of water (consisting of two atoms of Hydrogen and one atom of Oxygen). The term atoms refers only to elements.

Substances whose molecules consist of ions (atoms carrying an electrical charge) are called electrolytes.

The molecules making up matter are attracted to each other. However, the attracting forces between molecules tend to make them collide with each other, thus forcing them apart and creating an 'escaping' tendency which is directly influenced by *temperature*. As a result of these forces, the molecules of substances are in constant *random motion*. The physical state of matter, i.e. whether solid, liquid or gas, depends on the balance between the forces of attraction and the tendency to escape.

If the attractive forces are much greater than the escaping forces, the substance will assume a rigid, well-defined shape, i.e. it is a solid. If heat is applied to a solid, the escaping forces begin to overcome the attractive forces; eventually, the solid begins to lose its rigidity and starts to flow. In other words, the solid melts and enters the *liquid* state. As more heat is applied, the tendency for the molecules to escape from one another increases and eventually, the liquid boils and enters the *gaseous* state, where the molecules are so far apart from one another that the attractive forces have little opportunity to function.

Whether a substance is a liquid, solid or gas at *environmental temperature* depends on the balance of forces just described, since these forces are different for different molecules. The *transition* temperatures (the temperatures at which substances change from one state to another) for most ordinary substances are well outside the normal range of environmental temperature, but there are some familiar exceptions to this statement:

water is a solid (ice) below $0°C$

a liquid between $0-100°C$

a vapour (or gas) above $100°C$

ether is a liquid below $34.5°C$

a vapour (or gas) above that temperature.

Incidentally, a substance which exists in the gaseous state at environmental temperature is called a gas; if it is ordinarily a solid or liquid, but vapourises readily, the gaseous portion is called a vapour. Thus at room temperature, we would speak of oxygen gas but ether vapour.

The fact that substances are composed of minute, discrete moving particles makes it easier to understand that the molecules of one substance can mix with those of another. Thus, molecules of different gases mix readily because they are all so far apart. The molecules of a gas can also mix or 'dissolve' in a liquid; the less densely packed the liquid molecules, the easier is it for the gas to 'dissolve' in the liquid. Some liquids mix readily, others do not and this will be influenced by the *density* of the liquid (how closely the molecules are packed together).

Some solids will mix or dissolve readily in liquids, others do not. The ability to mix will depend on various factors but again, *temperature* plays an important part. In general, the solubility of solids *increase* with a rise in temperature, whereas that of gases *decreases;* this is because the higher the temperature of the liquid, the greater will be the movement of the gas molecules present in the liquid, so that they tend to escape from the liquid rather than remaining within it.

The weight of a molecule — the *molecular weight* — is the sum of the atomic weights of the atoms making up the molecule.

A molecule of *hydrogen gas* contains two atoms of hydrogen.

the atomic weight of hydrogen is 1
therefore the molecular weight of hydrogen is 2

A molecule of *sodium chloride* (common salt) contains one atom of sodium and one atom of chlorine

the atomic weight of sodium is 23
the atomic weight of chlorine is 35.5

therefore the molecular weight of sodium chloride is 23 + 35.5 = 58.5

When the molecular weight of a substance is expressed in *grams,* it is called *the gram molecular weight*

The gram molecular weight of hydrogen is 2 grams

of sodium chloride is 58.5 grams

of glucose is 180 grams

The gram molecular weight — or one gram molecule — of any substance *always* contains the *same number of molecules.*

Thus, 1 gram molecule of hydrogen gas contains the same number of molecules as 1 gram molecule of chlorine gas.

However, the chlorine molecule is heavier than the hydrogen molecule, so the same number of chlorine molecules weighs more.

1 gram molecule of hydrogen weighs 2 grams

1 gram molecules of chlorine weights 35.5 grams.

Looking at the statement the other way round, we can say that *equal weights* of two substances will *not* contain the same number of molecules

Physical Chemistry, Osmotic Pressure and Osmolarity

e.g. the molecular weight of albumin is 68,000

the molecular weight of glucose is 180

The albumin molecule is much heavier than the glucose molecule, so that 1 gram of albumin will contain fewer molecules than 1 gram of glucose.

It is often more convenient to express the concentration (or amount) of a substance in solution in terms of the *number of molecules* present. The actual number of molecules present is enormous, so for practical purposes, a terminology is used *based* on the number of molecules in 1 gram molecule of a substance — which we have seen is always the same, whatever the substance.

1 gram molecule of a substance (the gram molecular weight) contains 6×10^{23} molecules — over 6000 million billion

This basic number of molecules is called *one Mole*

A *molar* solution is one which contains 1 mole of the substance per litre of solution; and substances in solution are then described in terms of *molarity*,

e.g. the weight of 1 mole of sodium chloride is 58.5 grams (The gram molecular weight)

1 mole can be divided into 1000 millimoles, and

1 gram can be divided into 1000 milligrams

therefore a *millimolar* solution of sodium chloride contains 58.5 *milligrams* per litre.

The blood contains 330 mg of sodium per 100 ml of blood, which is the same as 3300 mg per 1000 ml or 1 litre

The molecular weight of sodium is 23

and 1 gram molecule per litre = 1 mole per litre

so that 23 grams per litre = 1 mole per litre

and 23 mg per litre = 1 millimole per litre

therefore 3300 mg per litre = $\dfrac{1 \times 3300}{23}$ millimoles per litre

= 143.4 millimoles per litre

Thus, the concentration of sodium in the blood is 143.4 millimoles per litre.

We have already seen that equal weights of different substances do not contain the same number of molecules — so that concentrations expressed in terms of weight are not always satisfactory. The concept of molarity provides a basis for comparison of the concentrations of different substances, whether they are present as molecules or ions, and whatever their weight.

Concentrations may also be expressed in terms of *Equivalent Weights*. This concept is particularly applicable to *chemical* behaviour and the way various substances react with one another. The Equivalent weight of a substance may be the same as its molecular weight; it may be half or less, due to the ways in which atoms combine with one another. Electrolytes, which are substances whose molecules are made up of ions — atoms carrying an electrical charge — are usually expressed in terms of Equivalent weights.

e.g. the Equivalent weights of sodium and chlorine are the same as their Molecular weights, so

the Equivalent weight of sodium is 23 grams

the Equivalent weight of chlorine is 35.5 grams

1 Equivalent may be divided into 1000 milliEquivalents

and 1 gram = 1000 milligrams

so 23 mg sodium = 1 mEq of sodium

35.5 mg chlorine = 1 mEq of chlorine

so 1 litre of a solution of sodium chloride containing 1 millimole (23 + 35.5 = 58.5 mg) contains 1 mEq of sodium ions and 1 mEq of chloride ions.

A solution containing 1 *Gram Equivalent Weight* per litre of solution is called a *Normal* solution, e.g. a Normal solution of sodium chloride contains 58.5 grams per litre. A common dilution is a one tenth Normal solution — written $\frac{N}{10}$ or N/10. Tenth Normal saline (or N/10 saline) contains 5.85 grams per litre.

N.B. 'Normal Saline' is *not* a Normal solution as far as Equivalents are concerned. It contains only 9 grams of sodium chloride per litre instead of 58.5 grams. The word normal is used here in a physiological sense and refers to the fact that the solution is *isotonic* with the blood.

In the blood, the concentration of sodium ions is
330 mg per 100 ml of blood
= 3300 mg per 1000 ml (1 litre)

Physical Chemistry, Osmotic Pressure and Osmolarity

the Equivalent weight of sodium is 23

so 23 mg sodium is 1 mEq

therefore 3300 mg sodium = $\frac{1 \times 3300}{23}$ mEq per litre

= 143.4 mEq per litre

the concentration of sodium in the blood may therefore be variously expressed as

330 mg per 100 ml – or 330 mg %

143.4 millimoles per litre (mM per litre)

143.4 milliEquivalents per litre (mEq per litre)

Physiologically, it is easier and more meaningful to assess deviations from the normal and to compare one substance with another, using mEq and mM rather than units of weight, since both chemical and numerical relationships are involved.

Osmotic pressure

If a solution of sodium chloride in water is placed in a tube which is dipped in pure water, the bottom end of the tube being covered by a filter or semipermeable membrane, the sodium and chloride ions and the water molecules will pass freely across the membrane until, at the stage of equilibrium, the number of ions and molecules is the same on both sides of the membrane. This process is called *Diffusion*.

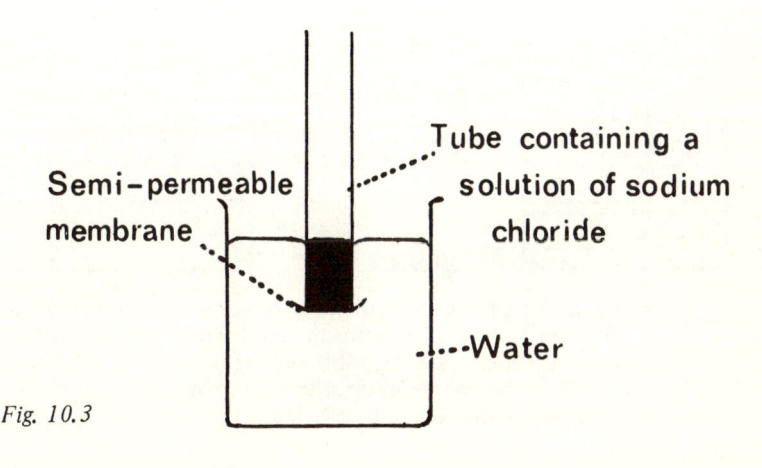

Fig. 10.3

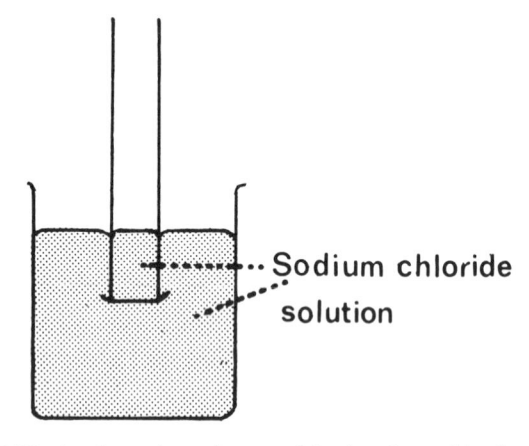

Fig. 10.4 Diffusion has taken place, and both tube and beaker now contain sodium chloride solution. Note that there is no difference between the fluid levels in the tube and the beaker.

If a solution of reasonably small molecules such as glucose is used instead of the sodium chloride, the same process of diffusion takes place. If however, a solution containing much larger molecules is used, e.g. albumin, the large molecules are unable to pass through the

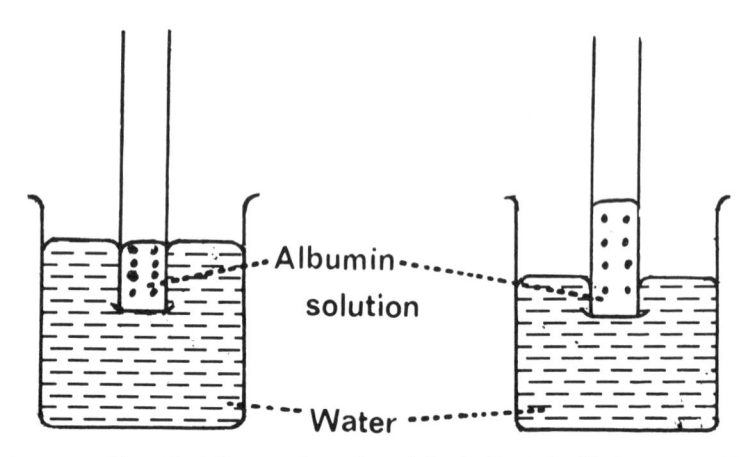

Fig. 10.5 Note that the *number of particles* in the tube (dots representing the albumin molecules) remains the same, but the *concentration* has altered. Water passes into the albumin solution so that the solution becomes more dilute; at the same time, the level in the tube rises while that in the beaker falls.

Physical Chemistry, Osmotic Pressure and Osmolarity 123

semipermeable membrane. Water molecules will pass across the membrane into the albumin solution however in an effort to attain equilibrium. The level of the albumin solution will therefore rise and that of the pure water will fall. See Fig. 5.

Water molecules will continue to pass into the albumin solution *until* the pressure exerted by the weight of the column of albumin solution prevents any further diffusion — and the pressure at this point is called the *Osmotic pressure* of the solution concerned. Note that the osmotic pressure of the solution is the same as the hydrostatic pressure exerted by the column of the solution, and can therefore be measured in cms, inches etc. Arranging the system so that it can be connected to a mercury manometer enables the pressure to be measured in mmHg.

The phenomenon of osmosis *only* occurs in the presence of a semipermeable membrane, when some particles are unable to pass across the membrane. For example, the osmotic effect of the plasma proteins is due to the fact that, under normal circumstances, they are unable to pass through the capillary walls. Ions and molecules taking part in metabolic processes pass freely across the capillary walls — but the movement of *water* molecules is influenced by the plasma proteins, which cannot pass. At the arterial end of a capillary, the blood pressure is higher than the osmotic pressure — so the water molecules are 'forced' out of the capillary. At the venous end, the blood pressure is lower than the osmotic pressure and therefore cannot prevent water molecules diffusing back into the capillary.

I think one of the reasons for confusion about osmosis in physiology is that the word *pressure* tends to conjure up a mental picture of an outward moving force — so when it is said that the osmotic pressure of the plasma proteins is responsible for the movement of water *back* into the capillaries, it would seem that an outward force has somehow turned into a negative, sucking-back, or attractive one. If we remember that osmotic pressure is the *potential* pressure that will be exerted by a substance in the presence of a semi-permeable membrane *if it is allowed to do so,* it might help to avoid confusion. As far as the plasma proteins and the capillaries are concerned, it is the *difference* between the blood pressure and the osmotic pressure which is important. The blood pressure is higher than the potential osmotic pressure of the plasma proteins at the arterial end of the capillaries. Since water molecules can pass freely across the capillary walls, they are therefore unable to remain within the capillaries, and are forced out into the interstitial fluid. At the venous end of the capillaries, the blood pressure is lower than the potential osmotic pressure of the plasma proteins, so it cannot prevent the water molecules diffusing back into the capillaries. One of the basic laws of chemistry is that particles in solution are always trying to achieve equilibrium. In physiology, many factors are acting to prevent them doing so — active metabolic processes, varying permeabilities of cell membranes etc. Ions and molecules are therefore constantly moving throughout the cells and fluids of the body — but their movement and overall concentrations are influenced and controlled by physiological processes.

The osmotic pressure of a substance in solution depends on the *number of particles* in the solution.

The gram molecular weight of all substances contains the same number of molecules, therefore molar solutions — containing 1 mole per litre — contain the same number of molecules. Molecules of electrolytes exist as their constituent ions rather than as molecules, so a molar solution of an electrolyte will have at least double the number of *particles* compared with a molar solution of a substance whose molecules do not exist as ions — although the number of *molecules* in each solution is the same. Molar solutions of non-ionising molecules have the same osmotic pressure; the osmotic pressure of a molar solution of an electrolyte will be double or more according to the number of ions in the molecules.

Solutions containing the same *weights* of different substances will of course have very different osmotic pressures. Osmotic pressure depends on the *number* of particles, so the heavier a molecule, the fewer there will be in a given weight of substance,

e.g. the molecular weight of glucose is 180

the molecular weight of albumin is 68,000

A solution containing 1 gram of glucose in 100 ml water will exert an osmotic pressure of 946 mmHg

A solution containing 1 gram of albumin in 100 ml water will exert an osmotic pressure of only 2.5 mmHg

Because the albumin molecule is much heavier than the glucose molecule, there are fewer albumin molecules *per gram* than there are of glucose — so the osmotic pressure will be lower.

Remember that electrolytes exist as ions rather than as molecules, so the osmotic pressure of an electrolyte will be higher than that of a non-ionising molecular solution. A molar solution of sodium chloride contains twice the number of particles than a molar solution of glucose so the osmotic pressure will be twice as high.

To indicate potential osmotic effects, the term *osmole* is used.

Referring back to the various ways in which the concentration of sodium as ions in the blood may be described, we can add those of the *osmotic effects,* and the list will read:

Physical Chemistry, Osmotic Pressure and Osmolarity

the concentration of sodium in the blood is 330 mg per 100 ml
- 143.4 mEq per litre
- 143.4 millimoles per litre
- 143.4 milli-osmoles per litre.

The units used depend on whether we are interested in weight, chemical combining activity, numbers of molecules or numbers of osmotically active particles.

The potential *osmotic* effects of particles in solution are described in terms of *osmolarity* and the concentration or number of particles present in the solution is therefore measured in *osmoles per litre*.

Remember that Molarity refers to the number of Molecules in a solution and that their concentration is measured in Moles or milliMoles per litre. Osmolarity, Osmoles and milliOsmoles refer to Osmotic effects and indicate therefore the difference between the total number of *molecules* and the total number of Osmotically-active *particles* present in a solution.

The body fluids and Osmolarity

About 60% of the body consists of water. The proportion varies with sex, age and build. The average adult male weighing 70 Kgm contains about 40–45 litres of water in his body. This water is distributed as:

Water in the cells — Intracellular fluid — (approximately 25 litres)

Water outside the cells — Extracellular fluid — (approximately 16 litres)

(a) — blood or intravascular fluid
(b) — interstitial fluid and lymph
plus water in connective tissue, bone, cerebrospinal fluid, gland secretions etc.

There is a constant exchange of water between the intracellular and extracellular fluid compartments. A sample of water labelled with an isotope is found to be evenly distributed throughout the body fluids within half an hour of administration — with the exception of less accessible water in connective tissue, bone etc.

Ions are present in large numbers in both the intracellular and extracellular fluids, and are therefore mainly responsible for the *osmolarity* of the body fluids, i.e. the concentration or amount of the particles in those fluids. In normal health, osmolarity is maintained constant within narrow limits, so the *total volume of water* in the body is largely controlled and maintained by the amount of electrolyte present.

Molecules such as glucose, urea and protein also contribute to the body fluid osmolarity. There is protein in the cells and in the plasma but very little in the interstitial fluid. The plasma proteins are unable to pass out of the plasma in any quantity since the walls of the capillaries act as a semipermeable membrane. The plasma proteins therefore exert an osmotic effect, which plays an important part in the distribution of water *within* the extracellular space.

Extracellular fluid osmolarity

Long-term maintainance of the composition of the extracellular fluid depends on the intake, absorption and excretion of electrolytes and their distribution throughout the fluid compartments of the body. The sodium ion has particular significance in this respect since it is the predominant single ion in the extracellular fluid. A sudden change in water balance or a disturbance in sodium intake or excretion will cause a change in the concentration or osmolarity of sodium in the extracellular fluid, and therefore of the total extracellular fluid osmolarity. Any change outside the normal range of extracellular fluid osmolarity is unacceptable to the body metabolism; if the sodium concentration in the extracellular fluid has been *reduced,* there is an increase in renal output of water and a shift of water from the extracellular fluid into the intracellular fluid compartment, in order to restore the osmolarity of the extracellular fluid. A *rise* in extracellular fluid concentration of sodium results in an increase in extracellular fluid volume, partly from retention of water and partly from a shift of water from the intracellular fluid to the extracellular fluid in order to restore the extracellular fluid osmolarity.

Thus, in order to maintain the osmolarity of the extracellular fluid compartment, there must be a change in the *volume* of that compartment until the various metabolic processes available have restored the situation to normal. The shift of water between the extracellular and intracellular fluid compartments results from the differences in osmolarity between them, i.e. it is an osmotic shift of water in response to a difference in concentration.

The effect of the plasma proteins

The *distribution* of water between the blood and the interstitial fluid is dependent on the plasma proteins; electrolytes play no effective part in the distribution of water on either side of the capillary membrane since the capillary walls are freely permeable to both water and electrolytes. The actual osmotic pressure of the plasma proteins is low — about 2 milliosmoles or 15 mmHg — but this pressure lies *between* the hydrostatic pressure of the blood at the arterial and venous ends of the capillaries. At the arterial end, the hydrostatic pressure is greater than the osmotic pressure of the plasma proteins, so molecules of water are able to pass out of the capillaries into the interstitial fluid. At the venous end of the capillaries, the hydrostatic pressure is lower than the osmotic pressure, and therefore cannot prevent water molecules passing back into the capillaries.

11

The E.C.G.

Every nurse will be familiar with the necessity for observing a patient's general condition and with taking the temperature, pulse and blood pressure. When a patient is very ill, not only may it be necessary to measure and record these things more frequently but it is often more important to notice changes as soon as they occur. This frequently requires more sophisticated apparatus to help the patient maintain his precarious hold on life. The word monitor means to warn, and this is just what the instruments are meant to do.

One of the aids most frequently employed is the *oscilloscope*. This instrument displays on a screen the pattern of waves representing the electrical activity of the heart which is called the Electrocardiograph or ECG.

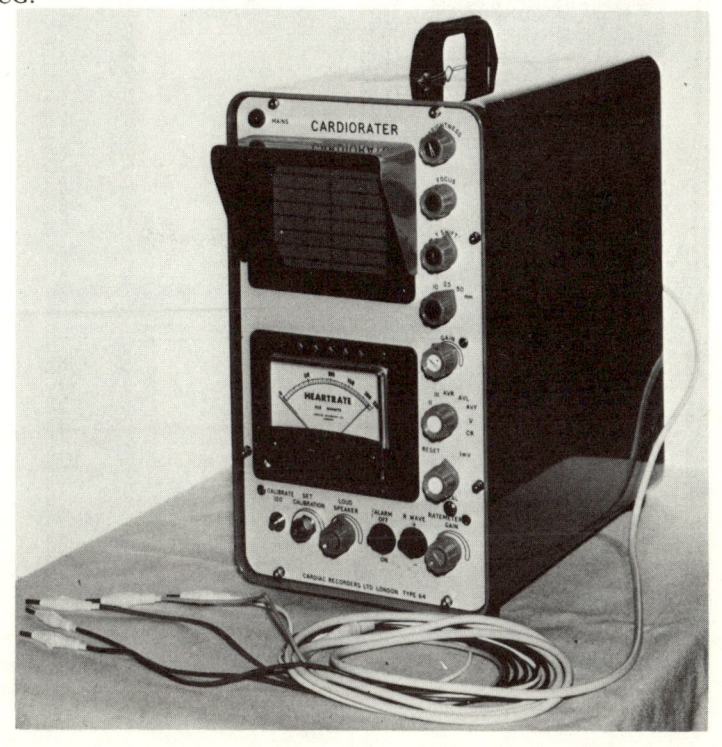

128   *Intensive Care for Nurses*

Oscilloscopes can also be used for displaying arterial or venous blood pressure. They are most commonly used as a visual aid, but it is possible to obtain from them both a permanent written record or a tape recording.

In the oscilloscope, the waves are traced out by a bead of light travelling across the screen, and the tracing fades away after a few seconds. Recently instruments based on the principle of TV have been produced where the tracing does not fade. The wave complex preceding each contraction of the heart appears at one side of the screen and moves slowly across, each new complex being added to one side of the screen and displacing the oldest from the other. The complexes form a strip, which may be stopped at any time to allow study of the strip and this 'memory-scope' as it is called therefore has considerable advantages over the moving light bead type whose tracing fades after a few seconds.

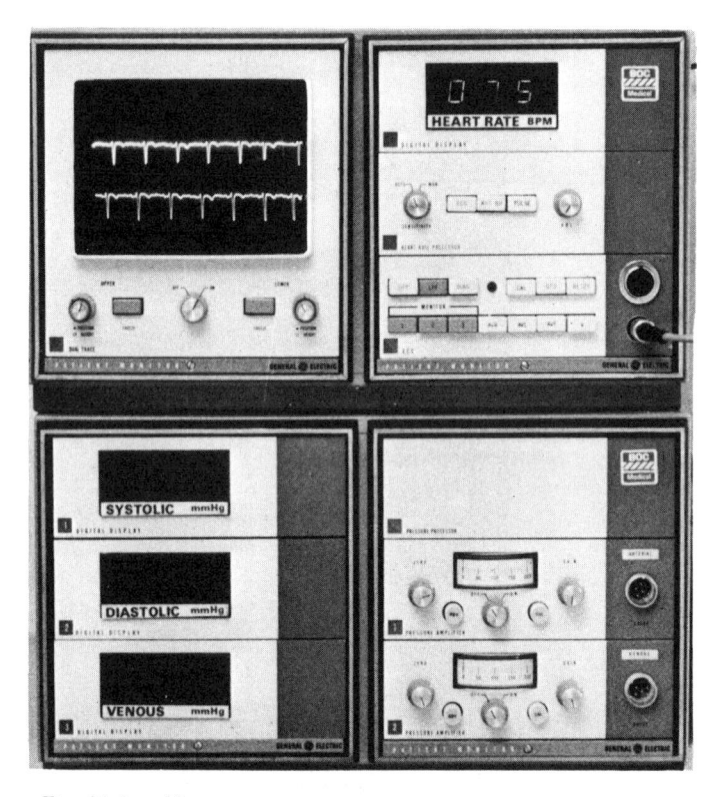

Fig. 11.2   Memoryscope

The Physiological basis of the ECG

All living cells have a positive charge on their surface and a negative charge within the cell. The two sides of the cell membrane thus have *polarity,* like the terminals or poles of a battery, and the cell is said to be *polarised.* The positive and negative charges on either side of the cell membrane are due to the presence of electrically charged chemical particles called *ions.*

Cations are positively charged ions; negatively charged ions are called anions.

Cations	sodium	Na^+	Anions	chloride	Cl'
	potassium	K^+		bicarbonate	HCO_3'
	hydrogen	H^+			

Although ions are diffusing to and fro across the cell membrane all the time, a greater concentration of cations (positive ions) is maintained outside the cell by an active metabolic process. There is thus an electrical difference — a Potential difference — across the cell membrane. Where there is a potential difference, a current can flow. The 'switch' for the circuit is the cell membrane. If the nature of the cell membrane is altered, charged ions which tend to be kept at one side or other of the cell membrane are able to diffuse across it unchecked. Their passage forms an electrical current and the process is called *depolarisation* of the cell. The movement of ions back across the membrane with the restoration of the potential difference is called *re-polarisation.*

The muscle fibres of the heart are cylindrical in shape and branch, uniting their branches with those of adjacent fibres. This means that a stimulus applied to any one fibre causing it to contract will eventually be conducted to every other fibre. This *conductivity* is a special property of heart muscle. There are further specialised muscle fibres which conduct a stimulus more rapidly than the ordinary fibres. They lie together forming a 'bundle' or conducting pathway known as the atrio-ventricular bundle or Bundle of His. Cold-blooded animals do not possess this pathway — and their hearts beat more slowly than those of mammals. Mammals are more active creatures and need a more variable cardiac output. One way of increasing the cardiac output is to make the heart beat faster. By having a fast conducting pathway, a stimulus arising in the right atrium will reach the ventricles more quickly and if the original stimulus comes more quickly the ventricles will beat faster also. The original stimulus arises in the sinu-atrial node or 'pacemaker' in the right atrium. An intrinsic ability to contract rhythmically is another special property of heart muscle. This is particularly developed in the collection of cells forming the sinu-atrial (SA) node, but it is also present in the atrio-ventricular (AV) node. Furthermore, without stimulus from either of these, the ventricles will beat rhythmically on their own, though at a very slow rate similar to that of cold blood animals. The SA nodes is supplied with fibres from both the *vagus* nerve and the *sympathetic* system, so that apart from its own intrinsic rate, the special cells comprising the SA node can be stimulated to initiate a slower or more rapid heart rate. From the SA node, impulses spread from fibre to fibre over the surface of the atria to reach the AV node. It is here that the atrio-ventricular bundle commences and conveys impulses rapidly to both ventricles.

The depolarisation and repolarisation of the heart muscle fibres produces the characteristic waves of the ECG tracing.

The Normal ECG

This consists of a series of waves which are labelled P Q R S and T. Each wave should start from a horizontal line and return to the same level. By convention, waves above the horizontal line are positive waves, those below it are called negative waves.

The P wave is the first wave and represents depolarisation of the atria. Depolarisation of the ventricles is associated with the series of waves known as the Q R S complex. R waves are positive waves. Any negative deflection preceding the R wave is called the Q wave. S waves are any negative waves following the R wave − or the major negative deflections if the other waves are inconspicuous or absent.

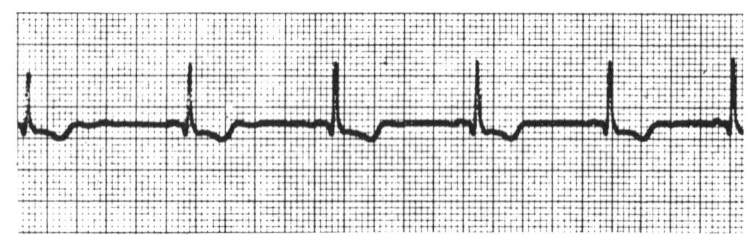

Fig. 11.3 Normal lead II

The T wave is associated with the repolarisation of the ventricles and may be positive or negative, according to the 'view' of the heart taken by the oscilloscope or ECG machine. The wave produced by atrial repolarisation is not usually seen as it is hidden by the Q R S complex.

Whether the various waves are positive or negative depends on the 'view' of the heart, so that the particular electrical lead is always stated, e.g. lead 1,

The E.C.G.

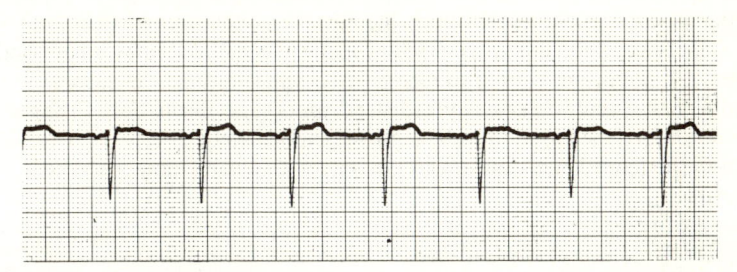

Fig. 11.4 Normal lead V_1

lead V_2 etc. This point is important, because some waves change polarity (e.g. a normally positive wave becomes a negative one) as a result of disease. No matter what the deflections are however, the nomenclature is always the same — any positive wave following the P wave (if present) is an R wave, any major negative wave in the Q R S complex is an S wave etc.
In lead 1, the P wave is normally positive, and there is usually a large R wave but only a small S wave.
In lead V_1, the P wave is negative. The R wave is small or absent but the S wave is large.

In order to pick up this electrical activity, contact must be made between the patient and the oscilloscope or ECG machine by means of *electrodes* and wire *leads*. It is important to make a 'good' contact. The skin should be sprayed and wiped with 70% alcohol to remove grease before placing a special low resistance jelly beneath the electrodes. Ordinary jelly such as K–Y should *not* be used as it is a poor conductor of electricity, and also tends to dry out more quickly so that contact is not so effective.

For diagnostic purposes, or short term monitoring, metal plates electrodes held firmly against the skin of the limbs by encircling rubber straps are most commonly used. Such straps could produce venous congestion if left on for a long time. In patients where monitoring is required for 24 hours or more, disposable electrodes with an adhesive plaster backing are safer. Small needle electrodes placed subcutaneously may also be used in the anaesthetised or unconscious patient.

For general monitoring purposes, the quality of the ECG is not so important as when, for example, an ECG is taken to assess the extent of a myocardial infarct. The nurse needs only to know, from some feet away, that there has been no change in rhythm or that the heart is still beating regularly. The experienced nurse will notice the onset of abnormal beats very quickly even though she may not consciously be looking for them. In the Intensive or Coronary Care Unit, sophisticated electronic apparatus is available which can count ectopic beats and recognise the onset of dysrhythmias, thus relieving the nursing staff of continuous surveillance of the monitor. However, although the nurse may not require to differentiate between all the abnormal tracings that can be produced by a damaged heart, it is important for her to recognise certain abnormalities such as ectopic beats, ventricular tachycardia and ventricular fibrillation. Changes in rhythm may be required to be reported immediately. If cardiac arrest occurs, the nurse herself must start treatment if valuable time is not to be lost.

ECG leads

ECG monitors offer a selection of leads and the pattern of waves displayed on the screen depends upon which lead is selected. Some tracings are smaller than others and their waves are less well defined. Leads II or V_1 are commonly used for monitoring purposes. Lead II provides a reasonable tracing for monitoring purposes but has the disadvantage of requiring the four limb leads. Lead V_1, obtained with a bipolar electrode so that only two leads are necessary, both on the chest, is now probably more commonly used in Coronary Care units; it has the added advantage that it differentiates between right and left ventricular activity in the presence of ectopic beats. Contractions induced by an ectopic focus in the left ventricle produce an R wave, whereas normally, there is a predominant S wave from the right ventricle lying underneath the bipolar electrode. Contractions resulting from an ectopic focus in the right ventricle will produce an S wave whose configuration is abnormal.

The size of the deflections can be increased by increasing the GAIN of the oscilloscope, but this also alters the quality of the tracing and can be misleading. ECG tracings will also vary according to the care used

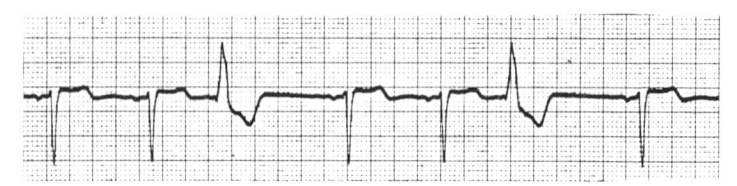

Fig. 11.5a Left ventricular ectopic beat. Lead V_1

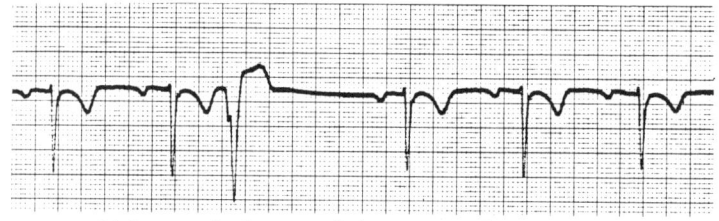

Fig. 11.5b Right ventricular ectopic beat. Lead V_1

in placing the electrodes, the size and shape of the patient, the presence of cardiac disease, and electrical interference from other apparatus. 'Mains interference' is a particular nuisance and may be present on all leads, often obliterating the tracing. In the majority of cases it results from poor contact at one of the electrodes. Common causes are

1) the jelly has dried out
2) an electrode is not held firmly against the skin
3) an electrode has become disconnected
4) one of the wires is broken.

In a few cases where there is a lot of electrical apparatus close to the patient, the interference may persist in spite of careful attention to the attachment of the electrodes.

The tracing can be kept in the middle of the screen by the use of the knob labelled Y axis. This knob moves the whole tracing up or down on the screen. The speed at which the bead of light (or the strip) moves across the screen can also be controlled. The knob may have a number of positions, e.g. 15, 25, 50 mm/second or it may merely increase or decrease the speed as the knob is turned, without there being any indication of the actual rate.

Analysis of the ECG tracing

1) *Count the heart rate*

> 5 large squares = 25 mm
> The paper moves at 25mm per second,
> therefore 5 large squares = 1 second
> and 30 large squares = 6 seconds.
>
> 30 large squares = 25 × 30 mm = 150 mm or 15 cm
>
> therefore the number of S (or R) waves in a 15 cm strip (6 seconds) multiplied by 10 = the heart rate per minute.

2) *Measure the regularity of the S (or R) waves*

> Regularity may be quite obvious. If there is any doubt, the distances between S waves must be measured by counting small squares. If the S-S intervals vary by more than *three small squares* (0.12 seconds) the ventricular rhythm is *irregular.*

3) *Examine the P waves.*

> A normal P wave preceeding each QRS complex indicates *sinus rhythm.* Absent or abnormal P waves with respect to the QRS complex indicate that the impulse has originated outside the SA node — i.e. an *ectopic pacemaker* is in command.

4) *Measure the PR interval.*

This is taken as the distance from the beginning of the P wave to the beginning of the *QRS complex*, since an R wave (a positive wave) is not present in all leads. The PR interval should be between 0.10 and 0.20 seconds, i.e. $2\frac{1}{2}$–5 small squares. Alteration outside these limits indicates *abnormal conduction* between the atria and the ventricles.

5) *Measure the duration of the QRS complex.*

If the distance between the beginning of the first wave of the complex and the completion of the S wave is greater than 3 small squares – 0.12 seconds – an *interventricular conduction defect* exists (bundle branch block)

12

The Coronary Care Unit

The aim of coronary care is to *prevent* death from the major complications of myocardial infarction by means of *specialised nursing care*. Originally, emphasis was laid on resuscitation – now it is aimed at prevention. Dysrhythmias are the most common complication of myocardial infarction. If the rate and rhythm of the heart can be continuously observed by electronic means, and highly-trained nursing staff are available to provide constant specialised nursing care, dysrhythmias can be treated as soon as they occur *before* the need for resuscitation arises. Even cardiac arrest is almost always preceeded by lesser, *warning* dysrhythmias.

If possible, all patients with a suspected myocardial infarct should be admitted to the coronary care unit, regardless of clinical condition at the time of admission, because the clinical course of this disease can be totally unpredictable. In the unit, they can be given the continuous monitoring, oxygen, appropriate drugs, possibly temporary artificial pacing and skilled nursing they require.

The average duration of stay varies from 3–5 days. Approximately 60% of deaths from myocardial infarction occur within the first three days and the system of coronary care has reduced this to less than 20%. This reduction has occurred predominantly in the numbers of deaths from dysrhythmias, and those from the other major complications, in particular cardiogenic shock and acute cardiac failure, have been less affected, Since the underlying causes of the circulatory failure in these cases are not always clear, it is more difficult to provide aggressive management of this problem. The routine use of frusemide however appears to be of help in preventing the development of heart failure.

On admission the patient is put to bed and allowed to rest propped up in the position most comfortable to him. There is no advantage in keeping him flat — unless he is very shocked. Even so, he should still have a pillow under his head. Nor is there any indication for placing him in the head-down position. This makes it more difficult to breathe easily, and although it will certainly increase the gravitational venous return to the heart, the heart may be unable to respond to this stimulus, so that the blood pressure and cardiac output fall.

The *ECG monitor* is set up and routine observations on heart rate and blood pressure are instituted.

Heart rate should be counted, using a stethescope over the heart,

$\frac{1}{2}$ hourly for the first 6 hours
thereafter hourly while the patient remains in the unit. He should not be disturbed at night however, unless absolutely necessary. At night, the rate may be checked from the monitor.

Blood pressure is at first checked hourly. If it remains stable after 6 hours, it is recorded 4 hourly, except during the night.

These observations will naturally be increased in the presence of complications such as unstable rhythms.

Oxygen is administered either by face mask or through light-weight nasal prongs, whichever the patient finds most comfortable and will wear continuously.

An intravenous infusion is set up, using 5% dextrose, to run 8—12 hourly as fluid intake should err on the side of restriction. Such a slow rate of infusion is facilitated by the use of a 'mini-drip' giving set.

Analgesia Pain and anxiety are hazardous to the coronary patient. They are liable to induce tachycardia (resulting in an increased oxygen consumption) and dysrhythmias. Dysrhythmias can interfere with the performance of the heart and may provoke cardiac arrest; an increased myocardial oxygen consumption is liable to extend the area of the infarction, since the cells in the immediate vicinity of the infarcted area are likely to die also if their activity exceeds their precarious oxygen supply.

If the patient is in severe pain, diamorphine (Heroin) 5 mg or morphine 5—10 mg can be given intravenously — slowly. If the pain is not completely relieved after 5—10 minutes, a further dose may be given — usually half the original dose will be adequate. Pethidine may be substituted if the pain is not severe.

Most units give routine sedation with diazepam 2—5 mg three times a day, initially intravenously and subsequently orally. This drug can be accumulative in its effect, particularly when renal function is impaired. Some patients become confused and mentally slow when given this drug and relatives should be warned and reassured that this is only temporary.

Administration of drugs

A patient who has a myocardial infarction may appear to have an adequate cardiac output as far as his systemic blood pressure is concerned, but in many cases, tissue perfusion is far from normal. Inadequate tissue perfusion means that absorption from muscle is reduced and drugs given intramuscularly will be less effective, and likely to accumulate. For this reason, all drugs are usually given intravenously until an efficient peripheral circulation has been restored. Routine insertion of an intravenous infusion on admission provides an immediate 'open vein' for drug administration, either in the normal way of treatment or during episodes of dysrhythmia or cardiac arrest. It also ensures a basal controlled fluid intake, *but* it must be remembered that when drugs are given via an intravenous infusion, a quantity of fluid is necessary to flush the drug into the circulation. Care must be taken to see that only the minimum of fluid is used for this purpose, otherwise the patient may be in danger of being overloaded with fluid.

Drugs given intravenously must be given slowly, in order to prevent overdosage. By giving a small dose and waiting for 1–3 minutes before repeating the dose, the effects of a drug, whether desired or adverse, are more easily controlled.

If heparin is used in the unit, it will be given intravenously in the infusion fluid until the patient starts mobilisation.

It is possible to combine the intravenous infusion with Central Venous Pressure monitoring (see Chapter 5). Most patients unless extremely shocked have reasonable veins in the antecubital fossa. A long catheter inserted here may be passed up the medial cephalic vein so that it comes to lie in the Superior Vena Cava or the right atrium. A 3-way stopcock placed between the proximal end of the catheter and the giving set facilitates

1) drug administration
2) monitoring of the pressure in the right atrium
3) the changing of giving sets.

Venous blood sampling via the catheter is not recommended unless absolutely necessary, particularly when the catheter is a very long one. A long, fine catheter means that it will take quite some time to withdraw an adequate amount of blood — and the blood will probably clot in the catheter meanwhile.

In some units, *left* atrial pressure is monitored in patients with cardiogenic shock. A special catheter is required, but the catheter is introduced via a peripheral vein in the same way as the catheter for right atrial pressure monitoring (see Chapter 5 on Venous Pressure Measurement)

Oxygen therapy

The amount of oxygen carried by the circulating blood depends on

    the haemoglobin concentration
    the percentage saturation of that haemoglobin with oxygen
    the cardiac output.

Both the oxygen saturation and the cardiac output may be considerably reduced by myocardial infarction. Increasing the inspired oxygen concentration ensures that the haemoglobin present is as fully saturated as possible under the prevailing circumstances.

ECG monitoring

The aim of ECG monitoring is to detect the development of dysrhythmias with the hope of preventing ventricular fibrillation. The risk of cardiac arrest diminishes rapidly during the first 48 hours following infarction although it persists for up to two or even three weeks. Apart from the danger of precipitating ventricular fibrillation, dysrhythmias can reduce the cardiac output. Anti-dysrhythmic drugs are frequently needed in the early stages but the majority of patients treated in the coronary care unit make a satisfactory recovery in response to rest, sedation and analgesia, together with the prophylactic use of anti-dysrhythmic drugs. A minority present with cardiac failure or troublesome dysrhythmias which require supportive therapy, synchronised DC shock or artificial pacing. If ventricular fibrillation does occur, it should be treated with immediate defibrillation, where possible.

On admission, each patient is attached to a monitor at the bedside. In most units, this ECG will be duplicated on a central screen together with those from other patients in the unit. This enables the nursing staff to observe the ECG of all patients in the unit at the same time without having a nurse at every bedside continuously.

The ECG may be traced out by a bead of light travelling across the screen, as in the oscilloscope. In the last few years, monitors have been introduced which are akin to television screens in that they show a whole picture at once, rather than building one up. The number of complexes visible at any one time depends on the width of the screen as well as the heart rate. The complexes form a strip which moves slowly across the screen so that any one complex is visible for a number of seconds. As the heart beats, the associated complex appears at one end of the strip and as the strip moves along, a complex disappears from the other end of the strip. The strip may be stopped at any time so that the ECG may be studied, and this form of 'memory scope' therefore has considerable

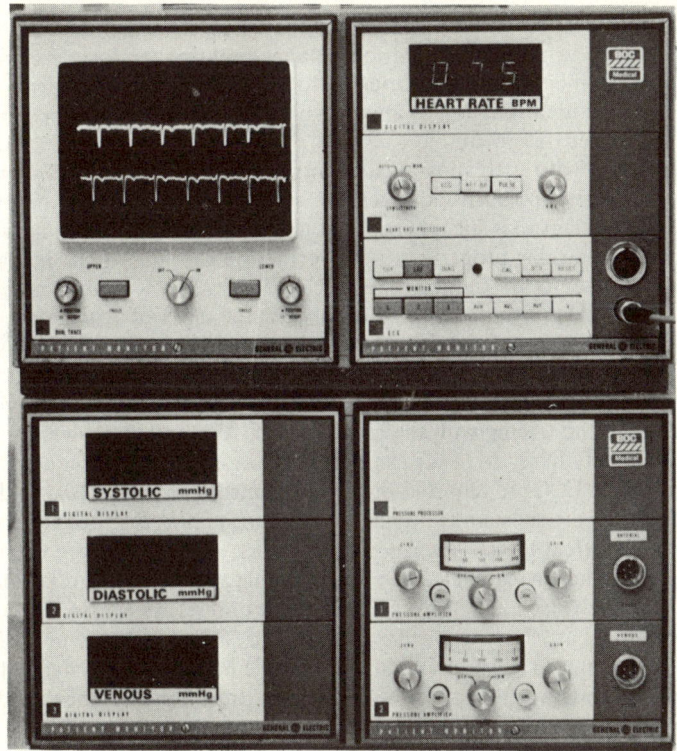

Fig. 12.1 Cardiac monitoring – Memoryscope at top left.

advantage over the simple oscilloscope whose tracing fades within a few seconds. *Written records* can be obtained when required. They can also be produced automatically in response to variations from the normal, or outside pre-determined limits, e.g. an increase in the number of ectopic beats, episodes of paroxysmal tachycardia, cardiac arrest etc. *Alarm bells, buzzers and lights* can be arranged to act at the same time. Tape machines can be provided to record continuously or on demand, as required. A tape machine is so designed that any previous recording is automatically erased from the tape before it passes across the recording head. For monitoring purposes, only a short period of recording time is necessary to provide a written record of the seconds leading up to a particular incident. On average, a recording/playback time of 40 seconds is quite adequate; the machine records for 40 seconds, erasing previous material as it does so, after which it starts again immediately for another 40 second period on the same piece of tape, and continues to do this indefinitely. These recordings are known as *'memory loops'*. The machines are set to *stop* automatically in response to a particular abnormality, e.g. ventricular tachycardia or ventricular fibrillation. The recording of the forty seconds *preceding* the incident is thus preserved to be available for subsequent study, and the identification of any provoking cause, as well as a possible guide to further treatment.

Familiarity with such apparatus renders it much less alarming. The more sophisticated the apparatus however, the more likely is it to 'give trouble' and it is important that the nursing staff who use it are able to appreciate whether it is working properly or not. Furthermore, senior nurses in many coronary care units are trained to use DC defibrillators on their own initiative, in order to reduce the time between the onset of ventricular fibrillation and attempted defibrillation. A sound knowledge of the ECG and the more common dysrhythmias is therefore essential.

When monitoring is started on the newly-admitted patient, the nurse should study the tracing with the medical staff. Abnormalities already present and any likely to occur can then be discussed. Any subsequent changes in the ECG are reported or treated immediately, according to the policy of the particular unit. Frequently, a *change in rhythm* does not significantly affect the performance of the heart; a badly damaged heart may however be having difficulty in maintaining an adequate cardiac output, and any change in rhythm can precipitate progressive cardiac failure. The occasional atrial or ventricular *premature beat* occurs in the normal heart. In a damaged heart, premature or ectopic beats are associated with the irritable state of the myocardium and may provoke recurrent episodes of ventricular or supraventricular tachycardia which can reduce the cardiac output. If ventricular ectopics are arising from more than one focus in the ventricle, then progression to ventricular fibrillation is almost inevitable. An *increase in pulse rate* may be due to pain or anxiety – or be an indication of incipient left ventricular failure. The coronary care nurse has to assess the ECG in association with the clinical state of the patient at the time, and then, within the instructions and policies of the unit, decide whether to report the situation immediately, initiate pre-arranged treatment, alter treatment according to instructions, or merely observe and wait.

The major complications of myocardial infarction

Dysrhythmia　　Greek dys – bad, therefore a bad rhythm; arhythmia (a – none) strictly means no rhythm at all. Dysrhythmias are the most common complication of acute myocardial infarction.

Heart failure
Cardiogenic shock
Thromboembolism
Pericarditis.

Heart failure

Myocardial infarction involves the left ventricle almost exclusively. Left ventricular failure is therefore more common than right ventricular failure, the latter being almost always secondary to left-sided failure. A decrease in the efficiency of the left ventricle leads to a reduction in the quantity of blood pumped out at each contraction — the stroke volume — and therefore the reduction in the cardiac output. Myocardial infarction decreases the efficiency of the ventricle by making it stiff and unable to distend normally, and the pressure in the atrium must be increased in order to fill the ventricle with blood during diastole. The change in ventricular compliance may be such that the ventricle is unable to fill adequately and as a result of this reduced filling and the decrease in efficiency of left ventricular function, the stroke volume and cardiac output fall. The rise in left atrial pressure caused by the reduced ventricular compliance results in a rise in pressure in the pulmonary veins, which, depending on the extent of the rise in left atrial pressure, will be reflected back through the rest of the pulmonary circulation. If left atrial pressure rises fairly rapidly, the hydrostatic (outward) pressure of the blood in the pulmonary capillaries will become greater than the osmotic (water-retaining) pressure of the plasma proteins, and causes pulmonary oedema.

Commonly however, there is only a moderate increase in left atrial pressure, resulting in the graduated increase in pressure in the rest of the pulmonary vascular system. This 'back pressure' creates a resistance which the right ventricle has to overcome. Initially, it will do this by increasing its force of contraction. An increase in left atrial pressure great enough to raise the pressure in the pulmonary artery — normally about 25 mmttg — will impede normal emptying of the right ventricle. The ventricular volume is further augmented by right atrial contraction during diastole — so the end — diastolic ventricular volume is increased, i.e. the ventricle becomes distended. If pulmonary artery pressure continues to rise in response to a progressively failing left ventricle, the right ventricle will become over-distended and the filling pressure will start to rise steeply, because of the stiffness of the wall of the ventricle. The increased force of the contraction will continue to maintain the stroke volume at this stage, and right atrial pressure, although raised in order to force blood into the distended ventricle, will still only be little above the normal limit. Ultimately however, this compensation is overcome. The ventricle becomes over-distended, it fails to maintain its stroke volume, and the pressure in the right atrium rises above normal limits, indicating frank right ventricular failure. The rise in right atrial pressure is reflected back through the venous system to the periphery, producing the picture of *congestive cardiac failure* — distended neck veins, peripheral oedema and an enlarged liver. The venous congestion is further augmented by disturbed renal function. *Left* ventricular failure is associated with salt and water retention which is due to a decrease in renal blood flow and an increase in the production of aldosterone. Retention of sodium and water causes a rise in extracellular fluid volume so that the circulating blood volume is increased.

Acute heart failure may develop immediately after myocardial infarction or over a period of days or weeks, depending on several factors. These include the extent of the myocardial damage and the ability of the heart to compensate for it. Left heart failure is by far the more common form of decompensation, owing to the fact that myocardial infarction almost exclusively involves the left ventricle. If the infarcted area is extensive, it is likely to produce a rapid rise in pulmonary venous pressure, causing pulmonary oedema.

Incipient left ventricular failure is associated with the stage of pulmonary *venous* hypertension, and the only sign may be an increased pulse rate in response to sympathetic stimulation in an attempt to counteract a fall in cardiac output. A chest X-ray will probably show dilated pulmonary veins.

If the pulmonary venous pressure continues to rise, small amounts of fluid are forced out of the pulmonary capillaries into the interstitial fluid surrounding the alveoli. *Interstitial oedema* is in most cases shown up on the chest X-ray, but seldom produces symptoms.

Clinical or overt left ventricular failure causes *alveolar* oedema. Since gravity affects the distribution of the flow of pulmonary blood within the lungs, it is not surprising that alveolar oedema occurs in the lung bases, where the flow of blood is greatest. The pressure of the blood in the pulmonary capillaries is normally higher in the lung bases than it is in the apices of the lungs; this postural pressure difference must be much less marked in the supine position, so the patient with alveolar oedema will probably maintain a more efficient blood-gas exchange if he is in the *upright* position and sleeps well propped up.

Since alveolar oedema reduces oxygen and carbon dioxide exchange, the patient is usually dyspnoeic. Rales can be heard at the lung bases and a third heart sound is frequently present, producing the distinct 'gallop rhythm'.

Marked left ventricular failure sometimes develops abruptly while the patient is asleep. Characteristically, the patient wakes 1–2 hours after falling asleep, complaining of suffocation and dyspnoea. Paroxysms of coughing may accompany the dyspnoea. The patient is obviously in acute distress and will sit up or attempt to get out of bed to reach the nearest window. The breathing is usually improved by the upright posture and the attack may subside within a few minutes; fear tends to increase and prolong the severity of the attack. These episodes of *paroxysmal nocturnal dyspnoea* represent acute decompensation of the left ventricle. Various precipitating factors are thought to be involved, including the horizontal position and frightening dreams.

Acute pulmonary oedema

This is the most advanced stage of left ventricular failure and usually represents a progression, or the culmination, of earlier signs of failure. The clinical picture is distinctive. There is acute dyspnoea, often with cyanosis. Respiration is noisy, and audible gurgling sounds can be heard as the patient struggles to breathe. There is often praecordial pain and incessant coughing with the production of frothy, often blood-stained, sputum. The patient is acutely distressed, with a rapid pulse rate and profuse sweating.

Treatment of acute pulmonary oedema.

1) Morphine is given immediately to reduce the distress. Morphine also reduces the respiratory rate and since the act of inspiration 'squeezes' blood out of the lungs into the pulmonary veins, a reduction in respiratory rate will tend to reduce the flow of blood in and out of the lungs and therefore the return of blood to the left atrium. The drug must of course be given intravenously as must every drug given to a patient with an inadequate peripheral perfusion.

2) Oxygen is administered, preferably by a close-fitting mask with a non-return valve, a reservoir bag and a high flow (8–10 litres per minute) in order to achieve as near 100% inspired oxygen as possible.

3) Frusemide 40 mg is given intravenously. This usually produces dramatic improvements within minutes, together with a copiuous diuresis. In theory, diuretics are effective because they reduce the intravascular fluid compartment by inducing a diuresis and therefore reduce the volume of blood returning to the left ventricle. The extraordinary rapidity with which pulmonary oedema is relieved suggests that other mechanisms are also involved.

4) Digoxin 0.5 mg diluted in 100–120 ml of 5% dextrose is infused over 2 hours.

5) Aminophylline 250 mg may be given intravenously over 10 minutes. It relaxes the smooth muscle of the bronchial tree and also stimulates the myocardium. It also produces renal dilatation and will potentiate the diuretic response to frusemide.

Cardiogenic shock

This is the most serious complication since probably 80% or more of patients who develop cardiogenic shock will die.

Although the precise cause is not clear, the effects are obvious — inadequate perfusion of vital organs resulting in death. Cardiogenic shock is the result of the progressive inability of the left ventricle to expel its contents effectively. It may be due to massive muscle damage, or involve the derangement of cardiac muscle metabolism resulting from myocardial ischaemia.

The clinical picture of cardiogenic shock

1) Mental state	There is mental apathy and lassitude. The patient seems dissinterested in his surroundings and stares into space. Alternatively, there may be confusion, agitation and restlessness.
2) Oliguria	
3) Hypotension	the blood pressure is 80 mmHg or less and there is a decrease in the pulse pressure. The systolic pressure generally falls before the diastolic pressure so that readings of 70/60 are not uncommon.
4) A pale, cold moist skin.	
5) Acute cardiac failure	The fall in cardiac output reduces the flow of blood to the myocardium, further embarrassing the ischaemic state. The patient with cardiogenic shock will almost always show evidence of failure — rales, a gallop rhythm, distended neck veins and the presence of dyspnoea.
6) Metabolic acidosis	The result of inadequate peripheral perfusion.
7) Hypoxaemia	

The prognosis is extremely poor.

Thromboembolism

There is an unusual tendency, and a high incidence, of intravascular clotting amongst patients suffering from myocardial infarction. The exact reason is uncertain. Most thrombi arise either in the deep veins of the legs — peripheral thrombi — or within the chambers of the heart — mural thrombi. If they break loose from these sites, the detached pieces of thrombus migrate as *emboli*, producing pulmonary, cerebral or peripheral embolism depending upon where they eventually lodge.

Pulmonary emboli arise almost always from the deep veins of the legs. They pass from the periphery through the right atrium and ventricle into the pulmonary arterial tree. Mural thrombi rarely cause pulmonary embolism since they are almost exclusively confined to the left ventricle.

The clinical picture really depends on the area of lung affected by the embolus. In many cases, there are no symptoms at all. Larger emboli are associated with sudden pain in the chest which is made worse on inspiration. There may be dyspnoea, cyanosis, cough, haemoptysis and a fall in blood pressure, depending on the area of infarcted lung. A massive pulmonary embolus obstructing the pulmonary artery produces sudden collapse followed by death within a few minutes. Occasionally, patients will survive for a longer period. It has been suggested that external cardiac massage tends to dislodge and break up the embolus in the pulmonary artery so that it passes on into the periphery. Where peripheral pulses and adequate oxygenation are restored within a few minutes following collapse and circulatory arrest due to acute pulmonary embolism, the patient has a faint chance of survival, but this is enormously reduced by the associated myocardial condition.

Consolidated areas of lung may be demonstrated on the chest X-ray, confirming the diagnosis of pulmonary embolism when the symptoms have been inconclusive. The ECG may show a distinctive strain pattern of the right ventricle which develops from pumping against the increased resistance created by the embolus.

Cerebral emboli arise from mural thrombi in the left ventricle. Embolism can occur very shortly after the myocardial infarct so it is not uncommon to find a patient admitted to hospital as a case of a cerebrovascular accident who has, in fact, had a myocardial infarct. The patient may have been alone when infarction occurred and the effects of the subsequent stroke will in many cases prevent the patient from describing either attack. A routine ECG on all patients admitted with a cerbrovascular accident can help to disclose a myocardial cause for the incident. Although most cerebral emboli do not cause sudden death, many patients will recover with a variable degree of function; but the combination of a cerebrovascular accident and myocardial infarction carries a poor prognosis.

Arterial emboli — Emboli from the left ventricle can pass on down the aorta to obstruct a peripheral artery, usually at a bifurcation. The most common sites are the iliac and femoral arteries, but any vessel can be involved.

There is acute pain in the extremity involved associated with skin pallor, coldness and loss of pulsations below the block. If the collateral circulation is inadequate, gangrene will develop unless the embolus is removed surgically.

Ventricular aneurysm and rupture

If the area of infarction is extensive, or healing is delayed for some reason, the wall of the left ventricle may weaken and bulge, producing a local aneurism. The cavity of the aneurism often becomes partially obliterated by organised clot. Ventricular aneurisms may be successfully removed with the aid of cardiopulmonary by-pass if the patient recovers from the myocardial infarct.

Rupture of the ventricle is the least common of the major complications of infarction, probably accounting for less than 5% of all deaths. Either the outer wall of the ventricle may rupture or less commonly, the interventricular septum. Rupture of the outer wall causes blood to fill the pericardial sac, producing *cardiac tamponade.* Death usually occurs within minutes. Rupture of the septum produces a left to right shunt and ultimately cardiac failure. It is associated with the development of a loud praecordial murmer and a rise in venous pressure. The prognosis is poor but surgical repair may be attempted.

Pericarditis

Pericarditis is commonly associated with myocardial infarction. There may be pain which may well be indistinguishable from the pain of infarction, but it is sometimes made worse by deep breathing. The characteristic friction rub is often transient and generally disappears when an effusion develops. A small effusion is often asymptomatic, but a larger one can cause pain, dyspnoea and orthopnoea, together with an irritating cough. An effusion large enough to interfere with cardiac function causes *tamponade.* This produces a rise in jugular venous pressure, tachycardia and a fall in systemic blood pressure. Pulses paradoxus — a diminution of the volume and pressure of the radial pulse during inspiration — may be observed.

Many units give Indomethcin routinely following myocardial infarction to prevent this complication.

Convalescence after myocardial infarction

The commencement and extent of mobilisation following myocardial infarction varies from unit to unit, but most units will allow the patient to feed himself, set up and move about the bed, read or listen to the radio and use a commode. Movement out of bed tends to be encouraged very much earlier than a few years ago and some units discharge patients on the 10th day for convalescence at home. Complicated cases will of course require longer observation and more cautious mobilisation.

Planned, regulated exercise is now believed to be of distinct value for improving the collateral circulation as well as for combating weakness and fatigue resulting from disuse of skeletal muscle.

The majority of patients who survive myocardial infarction are able to resume normal lives. Certain precautions will however help to prevent a recurrence of infarction and the development of chronic heart failure from residual myocardial weakness:

1) control of obesity
2) the treatment of any existing hypertension
3) regular sensible exercise
4) no smoking

13

The Treatment of Dysrhythmias Following Myocardial Infarction

The aim of treatment is to restore normal rhythm if possible and thereby
  prevent deterioration in the patient's condition
  prevent the onset of Ventricular fibrillation (VF) or Asystole

Ventricular fibrillation is precipitated either by a ventricular extrasystole or ventricular tachycardia. Extrasystoles should therefore be suppressed
  when they are frequent
    two or more follow consecutively
    the ectopic QRS complex occurs near the preceding T wave — commonly called 'R on T'
    the ectopic complexes are multifocal
    the patient has had previous episodes of ventricular tachycardia or ventricular fibrillation.

The prevention of *asystole* is less successful than the prevention of ventricular fibrillation. Asystole usually follows *massive necrosis* of the anterior wall and septum of the ventricles with damage to both bundle branches

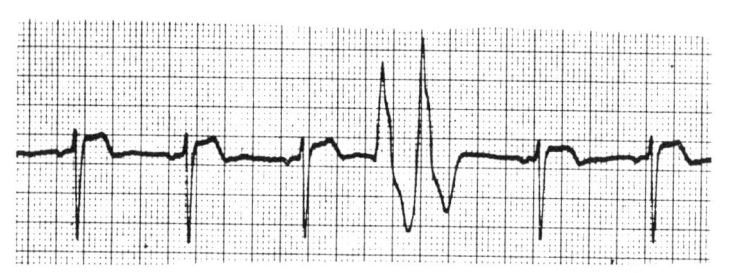

Fig. 13.1   Consecutive ventricular ectopic beats. The ectopic focus lies in the left ventricle as indicated by the R (positive) wave in lead V_1.

Treatment of Dysrhythmias Following Myocardial Infarction 149

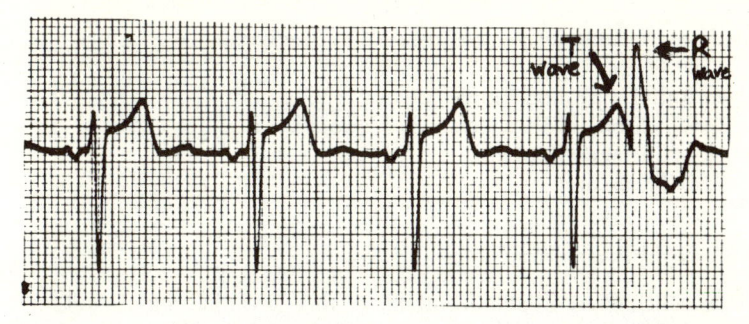

Fig. 13.2 'R on T' ectopic. Again, the ectopic focus lies in the left ventricle.

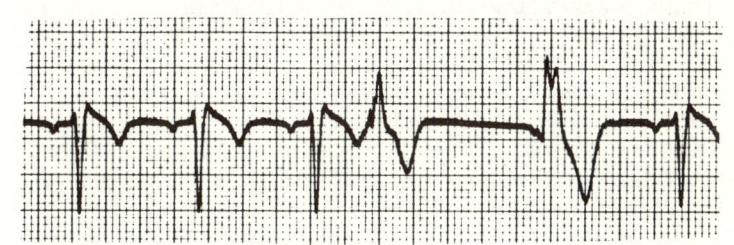

Multifocal ventricular ectopics. The shape of the ectopic QRS complexes is different, indicating different foci of origin within the left ventricle. The first ectopic beat is dangerously near the T wave of the preceding sinus beat.

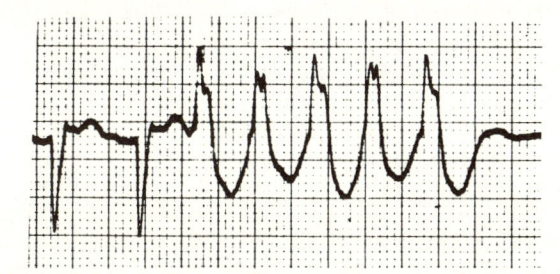

Fig. 13.3 A paroxysm of ventricular tachycardia.

travelling through the septum. Sometimes a subsidiary pacemaker does arise in the ventricle, but the resulting rate will be relatively slow and unreliable. An *artificial pacemaker* is therefore essential for survival, but the prognosis is very poor.

Inferior myocardial infarction may produce complete heart block, but the area of damage is less extensive and asystole is much less likely. Pacing is usually unnecessary; it may be required if the heart rate is very slow and does not respond to drugs, or if brief episodes of asystole occur.

Methods available for the treatment of dysrhythmias

1) Anti-dysrhythmic drugs
2) Synchronised DC shock — electroversion
3) Artificial pacemakers
4) Defibrillation

Anti-dysrhythmic drugs

Drugs which depress the inherent *excitability* of cardiac muscle will often suppress ectopic beats or paroxysmal tachycardia. Such drugs must be used cautiously however. Many cause depression of *conduction* either in the conducting system in general or in the atrio-ventricular node in particular. They may also reduce the ability of the myocardial fibres to shorten (or reduce their length) — i.e. they may reduce the *contractility,* and therefore the efficiency, of the heart muscle. If there is a large area of damaged heart muscle and the patient is on the verge of heart failure, any reduction in contractility may potentiate the failure and lead to a reduction in cardiac output.

Lignocaine in moderate doses will decrease the excitability of the myocardium without undue effect on conduction and contractility. Up to 200 mg may be given intravenously as a single dose and if effective, an intravenous infusion may be then employed to maintain control. Lignocaine is relatively safe and is probably the first drug of choice in the treatment of ventricular ectopics. It is unfortunately not always effective.

Bretylium tosylate may be successful where lignocaine has failed. It tends to suppress recurrent ventricular ectopic activity — but it also has a depressing effect on the myocardium.

Phenytoin (Epanutin) This is a useful drug for the treatment of ectopic beats but its action is somewhat unpredictable. Contractility is little affected, however.

Practolol blocks the beta (β) receptors of the adrenergic or sympathetic system. Anxiety is a potent cause of dysrhythmias and by reducing sympathetic tone, practalol indirectly helps to suppress ventricular ectopics. However, if myocardial function is already impaired by infarction, then the slowing of the heart rate by β blockade may well precipitate a considerable, possibly dangerous, fall in cardiac output.

Procaineamide is a general depressant, reducing excitability, conductivity and contractility, as well as pacemaker activity. It should be used very cautiously if there is any degree of atrio-ventricular (AV) block. The block will tend to be enhanced by the drug and conduction may then be so delayed that few stimuli reach the ventricles. Since excitability is also depressed, the ventricles may be unable to respond with their own intrinsic slow rhythm and *asystole* occurs. It is of value in treating patients who have had previous episodes of ventricular fibrillation, but it requires 3 hourly administration by mouth to maintain an adequate level in the blood and a frequent check on those levels.

Magnesium sulphate This drug has been found to have a general antidysrhythmic action. It is said not to depress the conducting system.

Atropine should be given where the heart rate is slow, as bradycardia favours the emergence of ectopic pacemakers. Provided that there is a response to the drug, it may be given regularly in order to maintain an adequate heart rate. If there is no response following a initial total dose of 3.0 mg, then artificial pacing may be required. Atropine increases the heart rate by blocking the effect of the vagus nerve on the pacemaker and the AV node.

If the bradycardia is due to myocardial damage rather than vagal activity then atropine is unlikely to produce an increase in rate.

Digitalis increases contractility and excitability but reduces conduction through the AV node. It also has a cholinergic action and therefore increases vagal tone. In adequate doses it slows the heart rate and improves the performance of the heart. Overdosage will cause bradycardia together with a tendency to ventricular ectopic beats, due to the increased excitability of the myocardium produced by the drug.

Synchronised DC (Direct Current) shock — Electroversion

When the heart is fibrillating, the passage of an electric current through the body causes the polarity of every myocardial fibre to change at the same time. As a result, every fibre is refractory to further stimulus until repolarisation has occured; after which the pacemaker will usually initiate sinus rhythm.

When the heart is *not* fibrillating, it is possible for an electrical discharge to *produce* ventricular fibrillation, if the discharge occurs just before the T wave. Repolarisation takes a definitive time to be completed so some fibres will be repolarised and ready to contract before others. An electrical stimulus applied at this time can therefore produce unco-ordinated muscle activity — i.e. VF.

Ventricular tachycardia is frequently a prelude to ventricular fibrillation. It can be interrupted with a DC shock, following which normal sinus rhythm will usually commence. With such a rapid ventricular rate, it is more than likely that a DC shock would be applied at the critical moment in the cardiac cycle and produce VF. In order to prevent this happening, a DC defibrillator can be made to synchronise its discharge with the R (or S) wave. This is known as synchronised DC shock or electroversion. It is used to treat sustained tachycardias that fail to respond to drug therapy or any dysrhythmias associated with a diminished cardiac output.

Artificial pacemakers

A variety of pacemakers are available, both temporary and permanent. In the coronary care unit, an *intravenous electrode* is the form most commonly used for temporary pacing. The electrode is introduced into a peripheral vein and passed up the vein so that its tip comes to lie in the heart. The tip may be left in the atrium for atrial pacing or passed on through the tricuspid valve into the right ventricle if ventricular pacing is required.

The insertion of the electrode may be done at the bedside. The subclavian vein is now commonly used, being cannulated percutaneously under local anaesthesia. Sedation is helpful. A small image intensifier designed specially for coronary care units is used to demonstrate the position of the radio-opaque electrode.

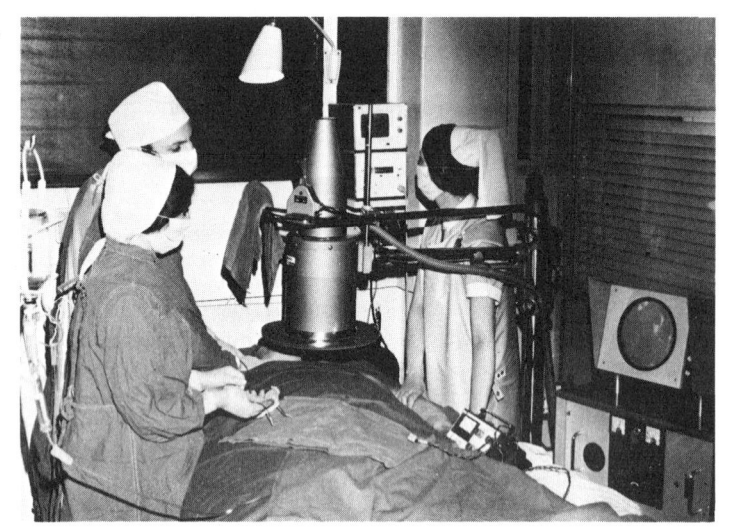

Fig. 13.4   Using the image intensifier in the Coronary Care Unit. The nurse on the right of the picture is watching the ECG monitor; the registrar inserting the pacing electrode is watching the X-ray screen.

Manipulation of the electrode will inevitably bring its tip intermittently against the walls of the heart, and this can provoke ectopic beats. If the myocardium is highly irritable, VF may occur. ECG monitoring is mandatory and a defibrillator must be available.

Atrial pacing may be used where atropine and isoprenaline have proved ineffective in treating sinus bradycardia, or to 'pace out' ventricular ectopic beats which do not respond to drug therapy. The faster the heart rate, the greater the possibility of the heart being refractory when an ectopic stimulus arrives. Using a pacemaker to produce an atrial rate of 90 or more will often pace out ectopic beats in this way. Atrial pacing is less likely to succeed when the ectopic beats are mutifocal.

Ventricular pacing is used where there is conduction block associated with an inadequate cardiac output, when episodes of asystole occur in complete heart block or, as a desperate measure, in persistent asystole. It may also be used to increase the heart rate to suppress ventricular ectopic activity — overdrive pacing. Some units have a policy of prophylactic pacing in all patients who develop an interventricular conduction block following myocardial infarction — in such cases, a fall in cardiac output or episodes of asystole will not be seen.

The artificial stimulus may be altered both in rate and in strength. When the electrode has been manipulated into place, the rate is set to the desired frequency and (in pacemakers generally in use in Britain) the voltage altered so that every stimulus produces a response from the heart.

Whether the pacemaker is set to the Demand or Continuous position depends on the clinical situation. Demand pacing means that the artificial stimulus is supplied only if the heart fails to beat, and usually this is arranged to occur after an appropriate delay. The time of this delay depends, (for a variety of reasons), on the setting of the demand rate. If the heart rate is too slow due to sinus bradycardia or conduction block, or if there is persistent asystole, then the artificial stimulus must be supplied continuously. Similarly, if overdrive pacing is being used to eliminate ventricular ectopics, then the pacemaker rate must be set to provide its stimulus consistantly at a rate faster than that of the natural pacemaker.

Dysrhythmias following myocardial infarction are commonly only temporary. The risk of cardiac arrest from dysrhythmias diminishes rapidly during the first 48 hours following acute myocardial infarction but can still occur within the next two or three weeks. In uncomplicated cases the heart rhythm should be monitored continuously for several days; patients with persistent failure or those with troublesome dysrhythmias in the early stages will require care for a longer period.

Defibrillation

This is the definitive treatment for ventricular fibrillation (VF). The sooner a DC shock is delivered, the greater is the chance of a successful outcome. If the shock is delivered within 30 seconds of the onset of VF there is a reasonable chance of restoring an effective cardiac output without further treatment. In many cases however, this is not always possible. The longer the delay between the onset of VF and attempts at resuscitation, the less likely is defibrillation to be successful at the first attempt. In this case external cardiac massage and artificial ventilation must be instituted without delay, and steps taken to counteract the metabolic acidosis consequent upon circulatory arrest.

Continuous ECG monitoring helps to reduce delay since in many cases it provides a warning of impending arrest, e.g. an increasing number of ectopic beats or episodes of ventricular tachycardia. If senior nurses are trained in the safe use of defibrillators and the defibrillator is ready by the bed of the patient at risk, then the delay between the onset of VF and the delivery of a DC shock is reduced to a minimum and influenced mainly by the time taken to reach the bedside and charge the defibrillator. The charging time varies according to the type of defibrillator and the intensity of discharge to be used. For emergency situations, a rapid charge time is essential — not more than 12 seconds for the maximum output of 400 joules.

One defibrillator paddle is applied to the praecordium (the area over the heart) and the other, well to the left.

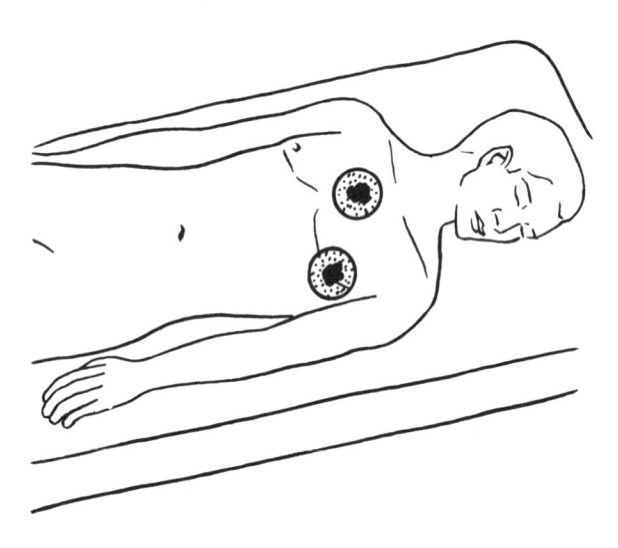

Fig. 13.5

Successful defibrillation is followed by a variable period of asystole. If QRS complexes do not appear on the monitoring screen within 3–4 seconds, a few sharp blows on the praecordium may stimulate the heart into activity. If not, then external cardiac massage and artificial ventilation must be started.

The return of co-ordinated electrical activity does not necessarily mean that the heart is contracting effectively. If there is no palpable radial or femoral pulse, continuous external cardiac massage is essential until a perceptible pulse follows each QRS complex.

Attitudes and techniques in the use of defibrillators vary considerably. Remember however, that a defibrillator is a potentially lethal weapon and it should be treated with respect. Carelessness could conceivably produce a second dead patient.

1) Nobody should be touching the patient or the bed when the shock is delivered — and this includes the person holding the paddles. For complete safety, one person should not hold both paddles, and rubber gloves should be worn.
2) Enough electrode jelly should be applied to provide adequate contact between the paddles and skin, but it should *not* be applied so liberally that it gets onto any part of the paddles other than their surface or so that, following successive attempts at defibrillation, the jelly from one area of skin encroaches onto the other. In both cases, arcing (short-circuiting) is liable to occur, which apart from being a potential source of danger to the operator and burns to the patient, is ineffective in treating the emergency.
3) KY jelly must never be used. It is a bad conductor of electricity and is likely to produce surface burns as well as being less effective.
4) A defibrillator should never be left charged for more than a few seconds. The person who has charged up the defibrillator must take the responsibility for checking that it has been discharged before leaving the machine.

14

Cardiac Dysrhythmias

Disturbances in rate, rhythm and conduction of the normal heart beat are called dysrhythmias. They may be considered in various ways.

1) The site of origin
    Sino-atrial node
    Atrium
    Atrio-ventricular node and junctional tissue
    Ventricle

2) The mechanism
    Bradycardia, tachycardia
    Flutter
    Fibrillation
    Premature beats
    Conduction defects

3) The effect of the dysrhythmia
    Minor effects — these frequently reflect irritability of the myocardium but seldom affect the circulation.
    Major effects — these may reduce the efficiency of the heart, give warning of impending danger, or cause death unless immediate resuscitation is carried out.

Cardiac Dysrhythmias 157

Analysis of the ECG

ECG paper is marked out in large and small squares.

   5 large squares = 1 second

   so 1 large square = $\frac{1.0}{5}$ = 0.2 seconds

There are 5 small squares in 1 large square, which equals 0.2 secs, therefore 1 small square = $\frac{0.20}{5}$ = 0.04 seconds

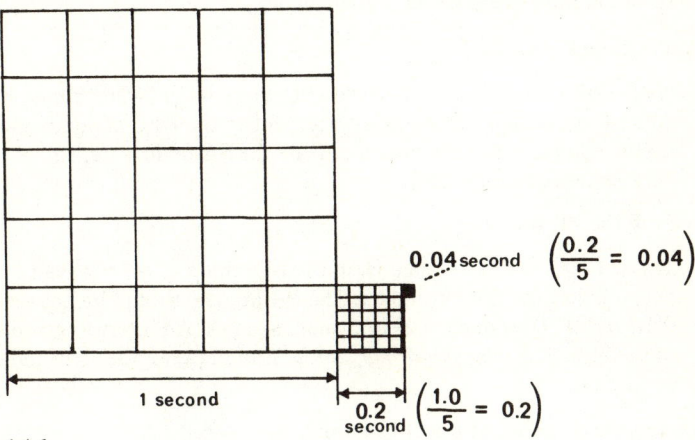

Fig. 14.1

Many papers are also marked at 3 second intervals along the top edge of the paper.

1) Count the heart rate.

   In 1 second, the paper moves 25 mm

   In 6 seconds, the paper moves 25 × 6 mm = 150 mm or 15 cm

   so that the number of S (or R) waves in a 6 second strip multiplied by 10
      = the heart rate per minute

   Alternatively, if 1 second   = 5 large squares

      then 60 seconds = 5 × 60 large squares,

         i.e. 1 minute   = 300 large squares

so that 300 divided by the number of large squares between S (or R) waves

= the heart rate per minute.

In both cases, irregular rhythm will create inaccuracy — but the first method is a useful and rapid way of calculating the heart rate.

2) **Measure the regularity of the S (or R) waves**

Regularity may be quite obvious. If there is any doubt, the distance between waves must be measured by counting small squares. If the S–S (or R–R) intervals vary by more than three small squares (0.12 seconds) the ventricular rate is *irregular*.

3) **Examine the P waves.**

A normal P wave preceeding each QRS complex indicates *sinus rhythm*. Absent or abnormal P waves with respect to the QRS complex indicate that the impulse has originated outside the SA node — i.e. an *ectopic pacemaker* is in command.

4) **Measure the PR interval.**

This is taken as the distance from the beginning of the P wave to the beginning of the QRS complex. The PR interval should be between 0.10 and 0.20 seconds — $2\frac{1}{2}$ to 5 small squares. An interval outside these limits indicates *abnormal conduction* between the atria and the ventricles.

5) **Measure the duration of the QRS complex.**

If the distance between the beginning of the first wave of the complex and the completion of the S wave is greater than 3 small squares — 0.12 seconds — an *interventricular conduction defect* exists.

Sinus Dysrhythmias

The SA node acts as a pacemaker to the heart because it normally discharges impulses at an inherently faster rate than any other part of the myocardium. If the SA node is depressed for any reason, other potential foci are able to replace it as pacemaker.

The rate of discharge from the SA node may be uneven, or may extend either side of the normal limits of 60–100 per minute. These variations produce 'sinus arhythmia', sinus bradycardia and sinus tachycardia. They represent the normal response of the node to the influence of the sympathetic and parasympathetic systems.

Sinus tachycardia may be a sympathetic response to fever, anxiety or physical exercise; it can also be due to reflex compensation for a decreased cardiac output following myocardial infarction. The development of sinus tachycardia in the patient with a myocardial infarct may indicate early left ventricular failure — which the rapid rate will tend to potentiate, since it increases oxygen consumption when the supply is already reduced.

Sinus bradycardia with a rate of 40—60 per minute seldom produces symptoms unless the cardiac output is reduced to the extent that there is an inadequate supply of blood to the brain or heart (producing syncope or angina). It is a potentially dangerous dysrhythmia because the slow rate encourages the emergence of a more rapid, ectopic, focus to act as a pacemaker. Sinus bradycardia should be treated if

1) premature ventricular contractions are also present
2) there are signs of a decreased cardiac output
3) the rate is 50 per minute or less.

The SA node may fail to discharge at all so that an entire PQRST complex is missed out; this may be noticed clinically as a dropped beat. On the other hand, an impulse may arise within the node but fail to activate the atria. This is called *sino-atrial block* as opposed to sino-atrial *arrest* where there is no impulse at all. Again, a dropped beat is associated with the absence of the PQRST complex. Sinus block and sinus arrest usually result from excessive vagal influence upon the SA node, but they can be due to ischaemia, or overdosage of digitalis or quinidine.

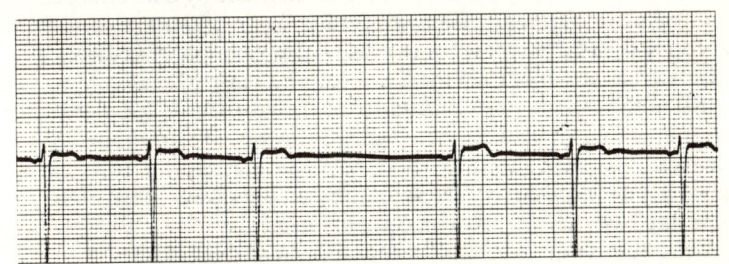

Fig. 14.2 The ECG shows rhythm at a rate of 60 per minute with normal conduction through the A—V node and the ventricles. A complete PQRST complex is missing.

Atropine will abolish the effect of vagal tone upon the pacemaker, and provided that there is a response, it may be given regularly in order to maintain an adequate heart rate. Initially, 0.3 mg should be given intravenously and repeated up to a total of 1.5 mg. If there is no response to this dose, the bradycardia is probably due to myocardial damage rather than vagal activity, and if an increased heart rate is necessary, artificial pacing will probably be required. Atropine will also be effective in cases of sinus block or sinus arrest where this is due to excessive vagal tone, but if they are due to myocardial disease, atropine is unlikely to produce an increase in rate.

Wandering pacemaker This dysrhythmia is again usually related to excessive vagal tone. The SA node remains the basic pacemaker but impulses occasionally arise in different portions of the SA node itself, or within the AV node. The shape and position of the P waves will reflect the site of origin of the impulse. Treatment is not normally necessary unless the AV node becomes increasingly dominant as a pacemaker. Atropine is usually effective.

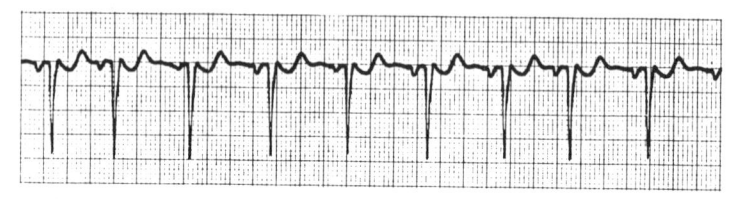

Fig. 14.3 The rate is basically regular, 90 per minute, but the P waves vary in size and shape.

Atrial dysrhythmias

These arise as a result of ectopic foci in the atrium displacing the SA node as pacemaker.

Ectopic means 'away from a place' and therefore by derivation, an abnormal place. *Premature beats* are cardiac contractions that arise from an ectopic focus. Premature (or ectopic) beats therefore result from a focus that has arisen outside the SA node. The ectopic focus may be located in the atrium, junctional tissue or the ventricle. When a premature beat is interpolated between two regular beats without disturbing the sequence, it is called an *extrasystole*. Attacks of rapid heart beats are known as *paroxysmal tachycardia* and are almost always initiated by a premature beat, i.e. one from an ectopic focus.

Atrial dysrhythmias are due mainly to increased myocardial irritability resulting from ischaemia or the effect of drugs. They are dangerous when associated with myocardial infarction because they are liable to increase the ventricular rate. Since myocardial infarction tends to reduce the efficiency of the heart as a pump, an increase in ventricular rate is likely to reduce the efficiency still further, as well as increasing myocardial oxygen consumption.

Premature atrial contractions (premature atrial beats, atrial ectopics)

The SA node remains the pacemaker, but the irritable atrium produces occasional premature beats.

Cardiac Dysrhythmias

The P waves of the premature beats are abnormal or inverted, but a normal QRS complex usually follows the abnormal P wave. There is a slight delay following the premature beat, known as a compensatory pause. This is due to the fact that the next impulse from the SA node, which would have caused the heart to contract, finds that contraction has already just occurred and that the ventricle is therefore refractory to stimulation. The subsequent impulse will be able to cause a contraction in the normal way.

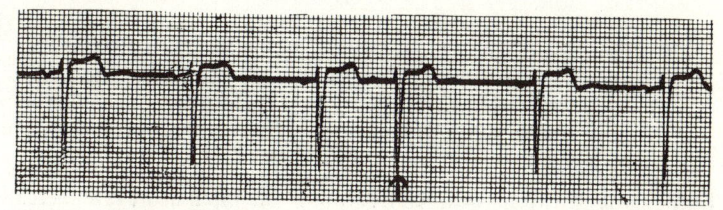

Fig. 14.4 Premature atrial beat. The rhythm is regular, apart from the premature beat which is followed by a compensatory pause. The P wave of the premature beat is positive whereas all the others are negative, showing that the impulse has not arisen in the SA node.

Treatment is not usually necessary unless the premature beats are frequent. This indicates considerable atrial irritability and the possibility of impending paroxysmal atrial tachycardia, flutter or fibrillation. Oral quinidine is probably the most effective drug in this situation.

Paroxysmal atrial tachycardia

Paroxysmal tachycardia in general is characterised by the following features;

1) it begins suddenly
2) the first beat of the attack is a premature one, i.e. from an ectopic focus
3) the beats are usually absolutely regular
4) the attack stops abruptly
5) attacks are often preceded by warning premature beats.

In paroxysmal atrial tachycardia however, it is quite common for the attack to subside slowly. The atria beat at rates between 140 and 220 per minute, and since the maximum rate of conduction of impulses through the AV node is about 220—240 per minute, the atrial contractions are usually all conducted to the ventricles so that the ventricular rate is the same as the atrial rate.

The P waves may be buried in the QRS complex or the T waves. If visible, they are abnormal. The QRS complex is essentially normal but may be widened. The rhythm is regular.

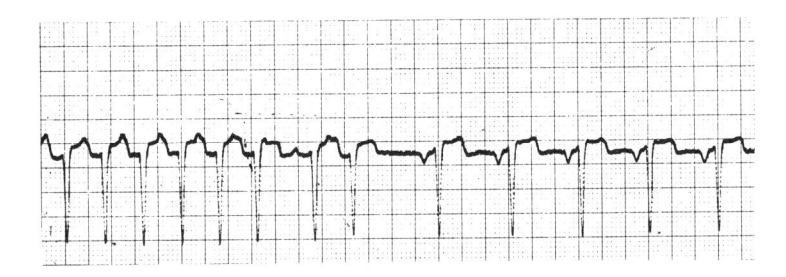

Fig. 14.5 Paroxysmal atrial tachycardia. The ventricular rate is regular, about 180 per minute. No P waves are visible, but the QRS complex is normal. The paroxysm stops after 6 beats, is almost provoked to recur by an ectopic atrial contraction (beats 7 and 8) but reverts to synus rhythm (beats 9 onwards).

In the patient with myocardial infarction, the rapid heart rate increases oxygen consumption, and this may provoke additional myocardial ischaemia and angina. The rapid rate also tends to reduce the cardiac output because the short ventricular filling time results in a reduced stroke volume. Under the circumstances, left ventricular failure is likely if the tachycardia is sustained.

Treatment

The dysrhythmia should be reported immediately even if it is relatively asymptomatic. It may cease abruptly without treatment; if not, reflex vagal stimulation through eyeball pressure or carotid sinus massage is often effective in terminating the attack. The carotid sinus lies at the bifurcation of the common carotid artery at the level of the thyroid cartilage. Turn the patient's head to one side and, with one finger, gently press backwards in the gap between the thyroid cartilage and the sternomastoid muscle. Gentle massage over the pulsating artery is then performed with the flexor surface of the finger, rather than its tip. If carotid sinus massage fails, practolol may succeed, otherwise a DC shock will probably be given. Digoxin is started immediately in order to prevent a recurrence of the dysrhythmia; troublesome recurrences can often be prevented by atrial pacing where the sinus rate is slow enough to allow an irritable atrium to provide a focus for ectopic beats. Where the dysrhythmia does not produce obvious symptoms, sedation with morphine is often effective.

Atrial flutter

An ectopic focus in the atrium stimulates the atria to contract 250–400 times a minute. The AV node cannot conduct such rates to the ventricles – only every 2nd, 3rd or 4th impulse will reach them, so the ventricular rate will vary with the degree of *physiological block* of the AV node.

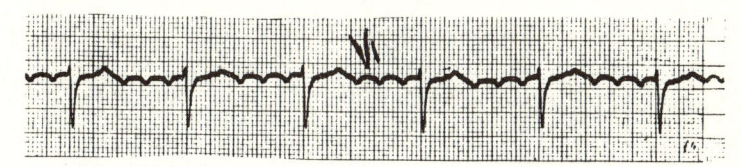

Fig. 14.6 Atrial flutter with a ventricular rate of 60.

The ECG shows characteristic 'saw tooth' or 'flutter' waves which are associated with the rapid atrial contractions. The ventricular rate varies from 60–150 per minute, depending on the atrial rate and the physiological block in the AV node. The QRS complex is normal, since conduction within the ventricles is unimpaired, and the rhythm is usually regular.

Treatment

Flutter may be treated with digoxin if the ventricular rate is between 100–130 and the patient's clinical condition is satisfactory. Digoxin slows the rate of conduction through the AV node and thus potentiates the physiological block, so that the ventricular rate is further reduced. If the ventricular rate is above 130 per minute or the clinical condition is poor, DC shock will be considered.

Both atrial tachycardia and atrial flutter are truely paroxysmal in that the heart can revert spontaneously to normal rhythm.

Atrial fibrillation

If an ectopic focus within the atrium discharges impulses at a rate greater than 400 per minute, the muscle fibres of the atria are unable to respond normally to such rapid stimulation; co-ordinated depolarisation and repolarisation cannot take place and the fibres contract individually, producing a generalised twitching of the atrial muscle. Rapid small waves called 'f' waves may be seen on the ECG. A proportion of these waves, representing the depolarisation of small areas of atrial muscle, will be conducted through the AV node to cause contraction of the ventricles. The pulse is therefore completely *irregular with a rapid rate* of between 80–160 per minute. If the AV node is damaged by infarction, conduction through it will be delayed, and in this case the ventricular rate will be *irregular and slow*. If conduction through the node is completely blocked, the ventricles will bear with their own intrinsic rhythm which is *slow and regular*, despite the presence of atrial fibrillation. A slow ventricular rate is

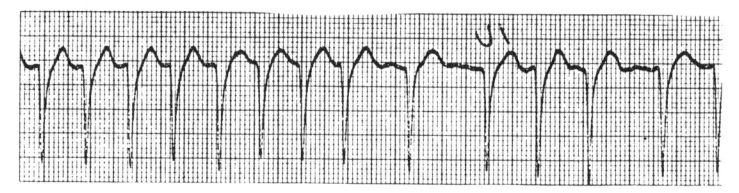

Fig. 14.7 Atrial fibrillation with a ventricular rate of 140. There are no P waves visible, and the ventricular rate is irregular.

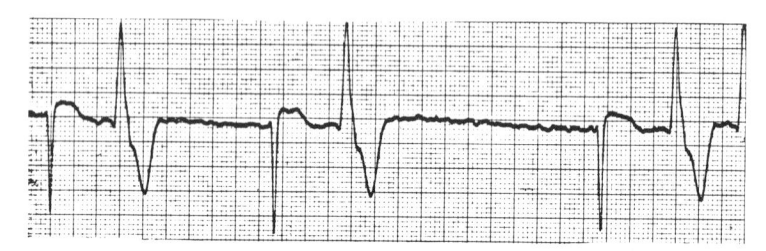

Fig. 14.8 The basic ventricular rate (consisting of the negative QRS complexes) is slow. The positive QRS complexes are ectopic beats arising from a focus in the left ventricle, creating an escape ventricular rhythm.

likely to encourage the emergence of ectopic foci. A ventricular rate greater than 100 per minute due to atrial fibrillation is called *uncontrolled* fibrillation.

Atrial fibrillation is frequently associated with myocardial valvular disease and under those circumstances tends to be permanent although it is occasionally paroxysmal. It is a serious dysrhythmia in myo-

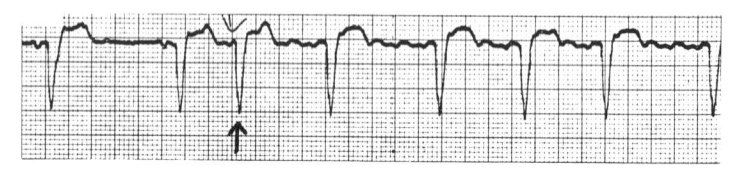

Fig. 14.9 The premature atrial contraction following two sinus beats (P waves followed by a QRS complex) sets off a burst of atrial fibrillation.

cardial infarction if the ventricular rate is high. If the ventricular rate is below 100, indicating a degree of AV block, treatment is not necessary, and both the fibrillation and the block may be expected to revert to normal. A ventricular rate between 100 and 130 associated with a good clinical condition should respond to digoxin 0.5 mg given intravenously in a small volume of infusion fluid over 2 hours, which may be repeated if necessary. If the ventricular rate is over 130 per minute or the clinical condition of the patient is poor, a DC shock will be considered.

Digoxin reduces the ventricular rate because it produces AV block, the extent of which varies with the level of digoxin the blood. By slowing conduction through the AV node, the ventricles are given a chance to relax and fill adequately before each contraction. This means that a reasonable cardiac output can be maintained in spite of the reduction in ventricular filling which follows from the loss of co-ordinated atrial contractions.

The development of atrial fibrillation encourages the formation of clots within the atria, with the possibility of embolism, so the patient must be observed carefully for this complication.

Junctional Dysrhythmias

The atrio-ventricular node (AV node) is composed of specialised tissue which delays the passage of impulses between the atria and the ventricles. It has no inherent ability to initiate impulses, i.e. it does not act as a pacemaker or as a focus for ectopic beats.

Areas of tissue adjacent to the AV node and the bundle of His are however capable of inherent spontaneous activity. These tissues are called *junctional tissues* and dysrhythmias arising from their spontaneous activity are called junctional dysrhythmias.

Junctional tissue as an ectopic focus

1) Impulses may arise in irritable junctional tissue producing *premature junctional beats* (junctional ectopics). The tissues may be so irritable that impulses arise more frequently than those initiated by the SA node, resulting in junctional tachycardia.

2) If the SA is depressed for any reason, the junctional tissues can replace it as pacemaker. The inherent rhythmicity of junctional tissue is slower than that of SA node, so junctional rhythm — or junctional escape rhythm, as it is called — is slower than sinus rhythm.

Junctional dysrhythmias, like atrial dysrhythmias, can affect the efficiency of the heart as a pump since they affect the ventricular rate.

Premature junctional beats

Isolated or infrequent premature beats have no significant effect on the circulation, but an increase in frequency should not be ignored.

The ECG will show

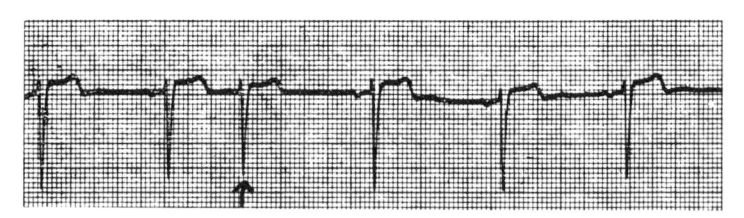

Fig. 14.10 Premature junctional beat. The QRS complex of the premature beat is the same as the other beats, but there is no P wave visible.

1) A normal heart rate.
2) Normal P waves, except for the premature beat.
   The P wave for the premature beat may not be visible; if present, it will be inverted, because the impulse travels retrograde from the junctional tissue to the atrium. It may appear immediately before the QRS complex or just afterwards, according to whether the impulse reaches the atrium before the ventricles or vice versa.
3) A normal QRS complex: it may be widened if the premature impulse stimulates the ventricles to beat before they have fully recovered from the previous contraction. A slight compensatory pause will be seen following the premature beat.
4) Regular sinus rhythm, except for the premature beat and its compensatory pause.

Treatment is unnecessary if the premature beats are infrequent, but an increase in frequency should be reported; if this dyrhythmia has required treatment with an intravenous infusion of anti-dyrhythmic drugs, the drip rate will be adjusted by the nursing staff to control the premature beats, according to instructions.

Junctional tachycardia may be paroxysmal, or established, i.e. persisting for several days. Symptoms are those associated with a rapid ventricular

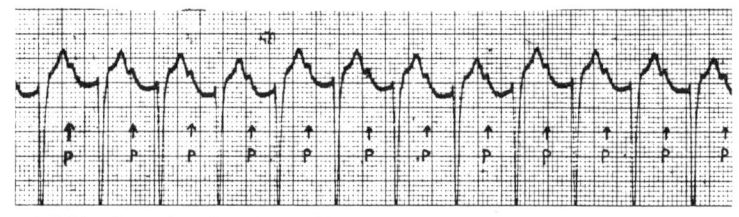

Fig. 14.11 Junctional tachycardia, rate 120 per minute. Inverted P waves, indicating retrograde conduction to the atria, are visible after the QRS complexes.

Cardiac Dysrhythmias

rate — palpitations and dyspnoea are common, and angina may occur if the tachycardia persists. The rapid rate frequently leads to a decrease in cardiac output, and in the presence of myocardial infarction, it can precipitate myocardial and cerebral ischaemia and left ventricular failure.

The ECG will show
1) A rapid rate of between 100—180 per minute.
2) A normal QRS complex.
3) Normal conduction to the ventricles: that to the atria is retrograde.
4) Regular rhythm.
5) The shape and position of the P waves, if visible, will vary according to the degree of retrograde delay imposed by the AV node. The waves are inverted. If the rate is very rapid, it is not always easy to identify the P waves and therefore to distinguish junctional from atrial tachycardia; in this case, the dysrhythmia is called a supra-ventricular tachycardia.

Treatment. Anti-dysrhythmic drugs may be tried initially if the patient is not distressed and the clinical condition is satisfactory, otherwise electoversion (DC shock) will be performed to terminate the attack; anti-dysrhythmic drugs are given in order to prevent a recurrence. Oxygen should be administered if the patient is distressed and a bolus dose of lignocaine 100mg may be given intravenously, according to previous instructions.

Junctional rhythm

Here the junctional tissue has replaced the SA node as pacemaker, usually because the SA node has been depressed as a result of excessive vagal activity, ischaemia, or digitalis overdosage. Since the inherent rhythmicity of junctional tissue is slower than that of the SA node, the ventricular rate in junctional rhythm — junctional escape rhythm — is slow, between 40—60 per minute. The slow rate predisposes to the emergence of other ectopic foci, particularly in the ventricle. Furthermore, junctional tissues provide a less dependable pacemaker than the SA node, and junctional rhythm can proceed to asytole.

The ECG shows
1) A slow rate of between 40—60 per minute.
2) P waves which are abnormal and inverted, because of retrograde passage to the atria.
3) A normal QRS complex.
4) Normal conduction to the ventricles but retrograde to the atria.
5) Regular rhythm.

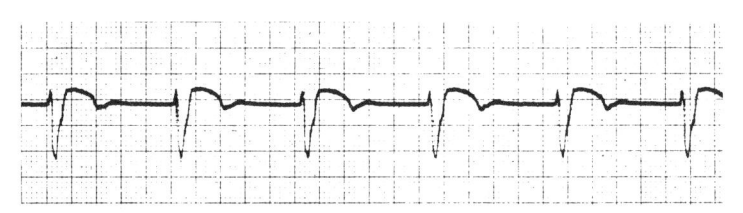

Fig. 14.12 Junctional rhythm — rate 60 per minute. P waves are not visible, being lost in the QRS complex.

Treatment

The development of junctional rhythm should be reported and the patient watched for the signs of an inadequate cardiac output or the emergence of further ectopic activity. Junctional rhythm is usually only temporary, and seldom requires treatment or produces symptoms, unless the ventricular rate is very slow. Any ventricular ectopics (escape beats) should be treated with lignocaine. Isoprenaline can be used to increase the ventricular rate but may well induce dysrhythmias at the same time; it also increases the oxygen consumption of the myocardium and can be difficult to manage as an infusion over a prolonged period. Ventricular pacing can also be employed to increase the ventricular rate; it has the advantage of overcoming the tendency to ventricular escape beats induced by bradycardia while being easier to control than an intravenous infusion; furthermore the ventricular pacemaker is instantly available should asystole occur.

Dysrhythmias Arising Through Abnormal AV Node Conduction — Heart Block

Impulses arise in the SA node and are conducted normally to the AV node; here,

1) they may be delayed — *first degree heart block*.
2) the time taken to conduct an impulse through the node may be so prolonged that recovery has not taken place before the next one, two, or even three, impulses have arrived at the node — *second degree heart block*.
3) conduction may be completely blocked, and no impulses pass to the ventricles. The atria and ventricles beat independently with their own inherent rhythm — *complete heart block*.

Ischaemia is the most common cause of heart block but it can be produced by digitalis or anti-dysrhythmic drugs. Heart block is not uncommon following myocardial infarction and is usually only temporary, but progres-

Cardiac Dysrhythmias

sion from the minor, asymptomatic first degree heart block to complete heart block with its potential dangers can occur, and very rapidly.

First degree heart block

The only abnormality is an increase in the PR interval which is greater than 0.20 seconds (5 small squares). There are no signs or symptoms associated with the condition and the diagnosis can only be made with the ECG.

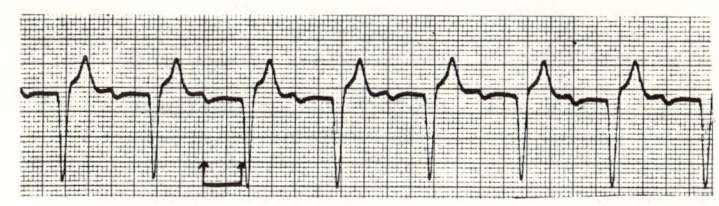

Fig. 14.13 PR interval. The ECG shows sinus rhythm with rate of 80. The PR interval is 8 small squares (0.32 seconds). It should be between 0.10 and 0.20 per seconds i.e. $2\frac{1}{2}$–5 small squares.

If the delay in conduction is moderate and does not increase, treatment will probably not be necessary. Increasing or markedly delayed conduction can be treated with atropine or isoprenaline intravenously, but the effect is unpredictable. A pervenous pacing catheter may be inserted at this stage in some units, but 1st degree block is not generally considered an indication for prophylactic pacing.

Second degree heart block

The time taken for an impulse to be conducted through the node is so prolonged that recovery has not taken place before the next one, two, or three impulses have arrived, and the ventricular rate is reduced according to the degree of AV block. Second degree heart block may thus be described as a 2:1, 3:1, or 4:1 AV block. Clinical signs are unusual and the patient often remains unaware of the dysrhythmia, unless the block occurs suddenly and the heart rate is abruptly reduced. The ECG shows:

1) a slow ventricular rate, one half, one third, or one quarter of the atrial rate.
2) there are two, three or four times as many P waves as there are QRS complexes.
3) a normal QRS complex.
4) every second, third or fourth beat coming to the AV node is blocked and never reaches the ventricles.
5) a slow and regular rhythm.

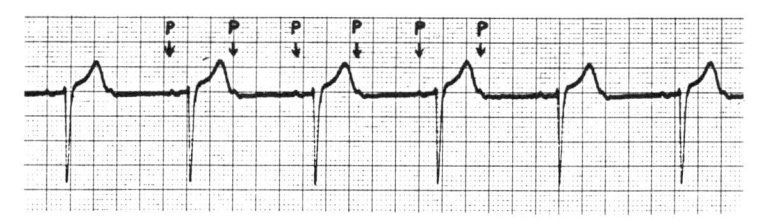

Fig. 14.14 The atrial rate is 120. The ventricular rate is 60. There is 2:1 atrioventricular block.

Treatment

Second degree block should be reported promptly since progression to complete heart block or ventricular standstill may be rapid. Atropine and isoprenaline may be given in an attempt to increase conduction through the node while preparations are made for inserting a pervenous pacemaker, and any intravenous infusion of an anti-dysrhythmic drug should be stopped.

Wenckebach phenomenon

This form of heart block represents progressive delay in conduction of impulses through the AV node. The PR interval becomes longer and longer until an atrial impulse arrives to find the node blocked so that the impulse cannot be conducted to the ventricles. Following the dropped QRS complex, the sequence is repeated. The Wenkebach phenomenon creates an irregular type of second degree block.

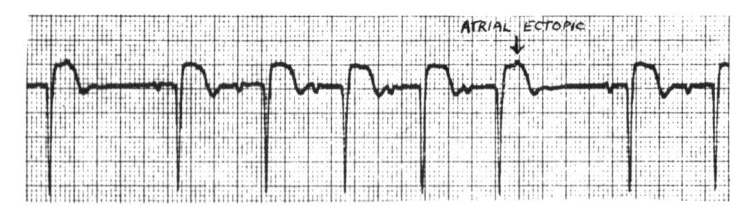

Fig. 14.15 The PR interval increases steadily from 5 to 7 small squares (0.20–0.28 seconds). In this example, an ectopic focus in the atrium then stimulates the atrium to contract — indicated by an inverted P wave on the ST segment. The ventricle is unable to respond, and a pause follows before the next P wave occurs.

Third degree or complete heart block

The AV node is unable to conduct any impulses from the atria to the ventricles. The inherent rhythmicity of the ventricles causes them to beat at a rate of between 25–40 per minute quite independently of the atria, which continues to beat at a rate influenced by the SA node. Independent or idio-ventricular rhythm is often an unstable rhythm; it may cease abruptly or may be replaced by ventricular tachycardia or fibrillation owing to the emergence of a faster irritable focus in the ventricle. The cardiac output is often inadequate for more than the smallest demand since the ventricular rate is fixed and faintness due to cerebral ischaemia is common. Extreme bradycardia or even ventricular standstill occurs quite frequently, producing syncope (Stokes-Adams attacks) unless measures are taken to prevent this. Attacks may last for a few seconds to 1 minute or more — recovery is unlikely after 2 minutes.

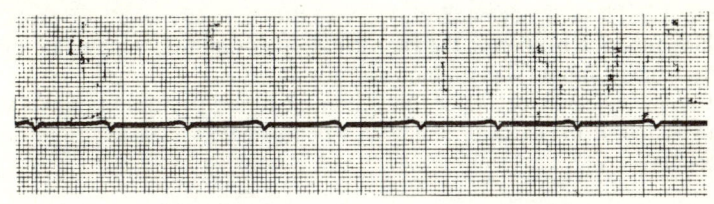

Fig. 14.16 Only P waves are seen. There are no QRS complexes, indicating ventricular standstill due to conduction block.

In complete heart block, the ECG shows:

1) a slow ventricular rate, commonly about 30 per minute. The atrial rate is usually normal.
2) There are more P waves than QRS complexes. The size and shape of the P waves are normal.
3) The configuration of the QRS complex depends on the site of the ventricular ectopic pacemaker and may be normal if the impulse arises close to the AV node.
4) There is no conduction through the AV node; there are two separate pacemakers acting independently.
5) Both atrial and ventricular rhythms are regular — but totally independent.

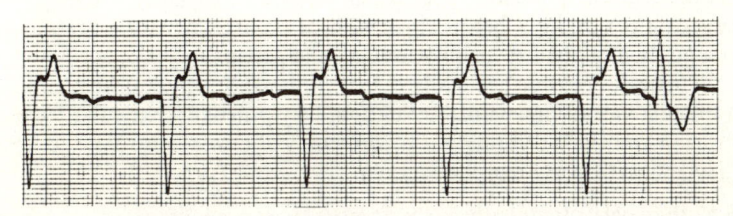

Fig. 14.17 The atrial rate is regular, approximately 150 per minute. The ventricular rate is regular, at 50 per minute, not including the ventricular ectopic beat. Note the P waves 'hidden' in the ST segment.

Treatment

This is essentially prophylactic, but complete heart block may occur before a pervenous pacemaker has been inserted. The dysrhythmia should be reported immediately and the patient watched carefully for the development of premature ventricular beats or ventricular standstill. If ventricular standstill occurs, a few sharp blows on the praecordium may stimulate the heart into activity; if not, external cardiac massage and artificial ventilation must be started without delay. The appearance of premature ventricular beats may be a warning of impending ventricular fibrillation and the defibrillator should be near at hand. If a pacemaker has been previously inserted and is of the demand type, it will automatically take over pacemaking function as soon as the ventricular rate drops below a predetermined value, usually about 60 per minute.

Complete heart block rarely persists and a return to sinus rhythm is to be expected. If the block does persits, a permanent pacemaker will be necessary.

Ventricular dysrhythmias

These are of three types.

1) *Premature beats* (ventricular ectopics) arising from an ectopic focus within the ventricular walls or the conducting pathway. They may be single, multiple or paroxysmal.
2) *Bundle branch block,* resulting from damage to the conducting pathway in the ventricle.
3) *Ventricular fibrillation* and *ventricular asystole* (cardiac arrest)

Premature ventricular beats

An ectopic focus in the ventricle stimulates it directly, causing a premature contraction. The premature beat is followed by a long delay — the *compensatory pause* — before the next beat occurs. Premature beats are commonly described as 'palpitations' by the patient.

Ventricular ectopic beats reflect irritability of the myocardium and, in the presence of myocardial infarction, may provoke ventricular tachycardia or ventricular fibrillation — commonly abbreviated to VT and VF. They are particularly dangerous when

a) they occur frequently — six or more times a minute
b) every second beat is an ectopic one — known as bigeminy
c) the QRS complex occurs near or on the T wave of the preceeding QRS complex — 'R on T'

Cardiac Dysrhythmias

d) premature beats arise from various ectopic foci — commonly called

multifocal premature contractions
multifocal premature beats
multifocal ectopics

Premature ventricular beats occur in about 80% of patients with myocardial infarction.

Features of the ECG

1) Rate — this is usually within the normal range of 60–100 per minute.
2) P waves — there is no P wave preceding the ectopic beat since this originates within the ventricle; normal P waves are otherwise seen if the heart is in sinus rhythm.
3) The QRS complex of the ectopic beat is always widened and distorted, since interventricular conduction is abnormal. The actual shape of the QRS complex depends on the site of the ectopic focus.
4) The time between the beat preceding and the beat following the premature ventricular beat is equal to two normal beats. A compensatory pause follows the premature beat.

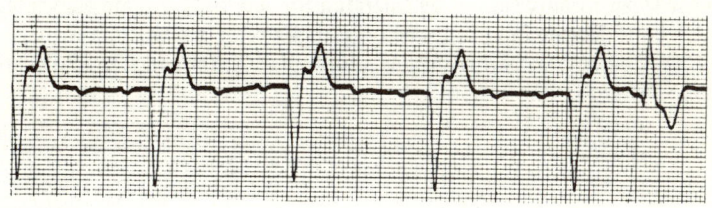

Fig. 14.18

Treatment

Lignocaine is the first line of defence. A bolus dose of 100–200 mg (10 ml of 1% or 5 ml of 2% contains 100 mg) is given intravenously and should be followed by an intravenous infusion to maintain control. A strong solution of lignocaine is necessary if infusion of a large quantity of fluid is to be avoided, and a 'mini-drip' is helpful here. The standard giving set delivers 15 drops per ml compared with 60 drops per ml in a mini-drip. 1 gram of lignocaine in a bottle of 500 ml 5% dextrose is a concentration of 2mg per ml — so an initial infusion rate of 1 mg per minute, using a standard giving set, would require a drip rate of 7–8 drops per minute. With a mini-drip, the rate would be 30 drops per minute — much easier to regulate and vary as necessary.

Lignocaine is rapidly broken down by the body, its effect lasting about 10–15 minutes, but the patient must be watched carefully for signs of overdosage. A high blood level will produce convulsions but these are preceded by drowsiness and usually, adequate warning of overdosage is given by muscle twitching, particularly of the facial muscles. If lignocaine fails to control ectopic activity, procaineamide or phenytoin may be considered, or atrial pacing.

Paroxysmal ventricular tachycardia

This may occur in short runs, stopping spontaneously after a few seconds, or it may be sustained for longer periods. The patient is usually aware of the sudden onset of a rapid heart rate and will frequently complain of dyspnoea, palpitations and pain in the chest. 50% of episodes may be expected to end abruptly without treatment; if the initial attacks are of short duration and the patient remains conscious, a bolus dose of lignocaine followed by an intravenous infusion may prevent further recurrence of the dysrhythmia. If the ventricular rate is seen to be accelerating or the clinical condition is poor, a DC shock must be given immediately. Where possible, 10 mg diazepam should be given intravenously beforehand.

The effect of ventricular tachycardia on the patient is closely related to the ventricular rate and the state of the myocardium. Ventricular rates of over 200 per minute cannot be tolerated for very long and are associated with a considerable fall in cardiac output. Extreme tachycardia with a rate of 250 or more is sometimes called ventricular flutter and frequently precedes ventricular fibrillation.

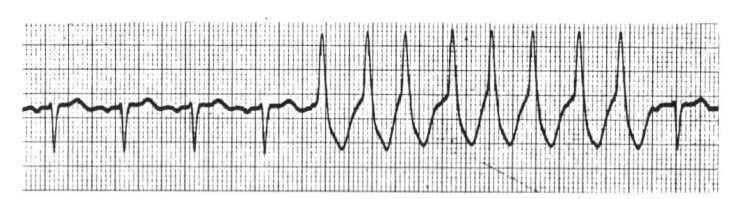

Fig. 14.19a Sinus rhythm is interrupted by a short paroxysm of ventricular tachycardia – rate 160.

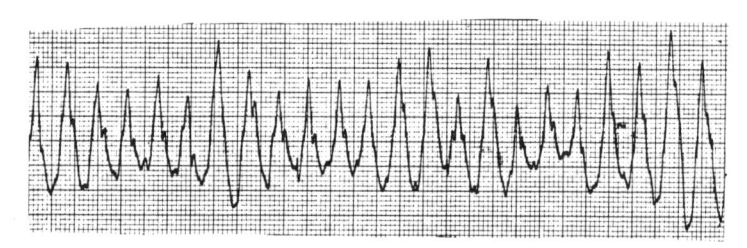

Fig. 14.19b Another example of ventricular tachycardia – rate 230.

Cardiac Dysrhythmias 175

Bundle block

Damage to the interventricular septum prevents impulses travelling along the ventricular pathway (the Bundle of His). The interruption may occur at any level in the bundle branches. The result is a delay in the time required to stimulate contraction of the ventricles, because the affected ventricle must be activated indirectly by impulses reaching it from the normally stimulated one. Occasionally, bundle block is complete, causing asystole, and ventricular pacing will be necessary either on a short term basis until healing has occured or, in some cases, permanently.

A full ECG is usually necessary to localise the postion of a bundle branch block, but its presence is obvious from the fact that the time for the QRS complex is greater than 0.12 seconds (3 small squares), and indicates damage to the interventricular septum.

The ECG in bundle branch block:

1) the rate is usually normal
2) P waves are normal
3) QRS complexes are always widened and distorted, being greater than 0.12 seconds (3 small squares)
4) Conduction is normal from the SA node to the site of the bundle block (i.e. a normal PR interval) but is abnormal within the affected part of the ventricle, thus causing the widened or notched QRS complexes.
5) Rhythm is regular.

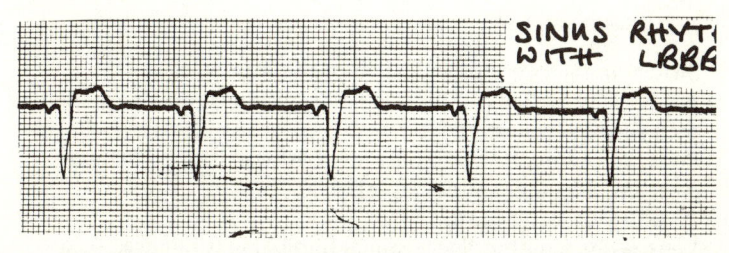

Fig. 14.20 The time for the QRS complex – normally not longer than 0.12 seconds (3 small squares) – is $3\frac{1}{2}$ – 4 small squares (0.14–0.16 seconds), indicating an interventricular conduction block.

Incidentally, the pattern of left BBB obscures the characteristic ECG changes of acute myocardial infarction. A patient with an appropriate history together with bundle block should be treated as a case of myocardial infarction until proved otherwise.

Bundle branch block causes no specific symptoms. Development of the block following infarction may indicate further spread of ischaemic damage and some units advocate the prophylactic insertion of an intravenous pacing electrode in these circumstances. The value of this technique is still debated, but it would appear to have a rational basis.

Ventricular fibrillation

The normal co-ordinated myocardial activity is replaced by totally unco-ordinated and continuous twitching of the individual myocardial fibres. The loss of co-ordinated contraction means that blood is not expelled from the heart and within seconds the patient loses consciousness.

The ECG is characteristic. The waves are haphazard, rapid and irregular.

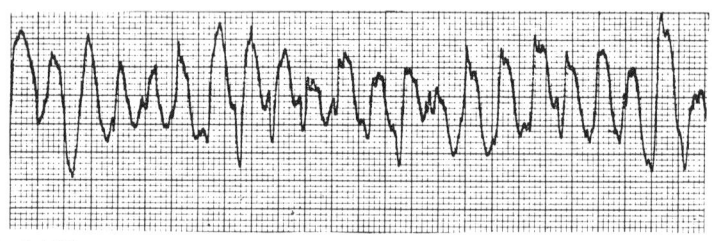

Fig. 14.21

Treatment

Immediate defibrillation.

Steps in defibrillation

1) Switch on the defibrillator and charge to 400 joules
2) Apply electrode jelly to the paddles, spreading it evenly by rotating their surfaces against each other.
3) Press the paddles firmly against the chest wall, one on the praecordium, the other against the left side.
4) Press the discharge button.
5) Look at the monitor. Successful defibrillation is followed by a variable period of asystole, after which spontaneous co-ordinated rhythm is resumed.

If the period of asystole persists for more than a few seconds, a few sharp blows to the praecordium will frequently stimulate the heart into activity. If this fails, external cardiac massage and artificial ventilation must be started without delay.

If defibrillation is effective, as shown by the presence of co-ordinated rhythm on the ECG, immediately feel for a peripheral pulse. Frequently, effective contraction lags behind the restoration of electrical activity, and

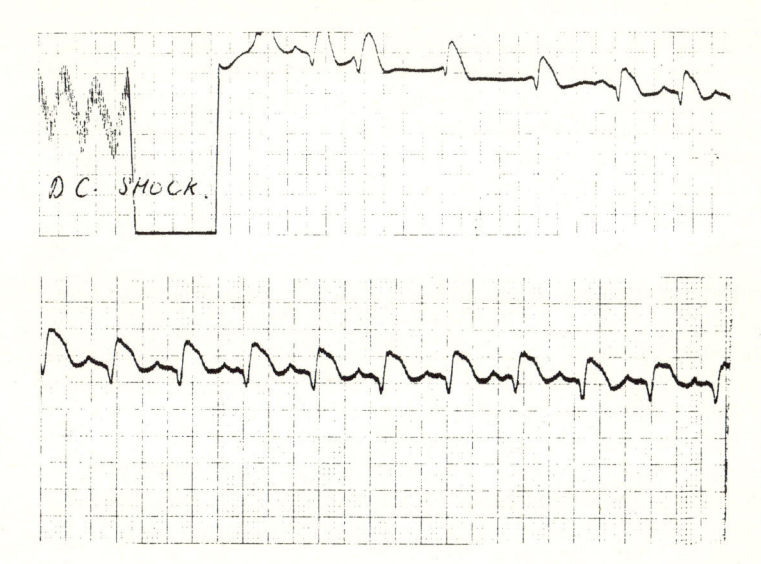

Fig. 14.22 Successful defibrillation. The two strips are consecutive. The ECG shows 'ventricular flutter' which inevitably proceeds to ventricular fibrillation. Sinus rhythm returns promptly following the DC shock, except for the 3rd and 4th beat. The QRS complex occupies more than 3 small squares, indicating an interventricular conduction defect.

cardiac massage is necessary to support the circulation until co-ordinated rhythm is accompanied by a palpable peripheral pulse.

Once the emergency is over, attention can be turned to the problem of preventing a recurrence. Meanwhile, it is important to make sure that the patient's clinical condition is satisfactory and that he is as comfortable as possible both physically and mentally.

If ventricular fibrillation persists following the first shock, a second should be given immediately; if this too fails, routine measures for the treatment of cardiac arrest must be instituted without further delay.

The successful restoration of a spontaneous heart beat is related to the time interval between the onset of fibrillation and administration of the DC shock. The longer the delay, the less likely is the outcome to be successful. This is partly due to the metabolic acidosis which builds up rapidly following circulatory arrest. If defibrillation fails in the first instance, 50–100 mEq of sodium bicarbonate should be given intravenously before the next attempt. Ideally, 8.4% solutions (1mEq per ml) should be provided in 100 ml bottles for this purpose but there are problems associated with this as special glass is necessary. There are solutions of 8.4% available commercially, but these come in 500 ml semi-rigid plastic containers; in moments of stress, it is quite impractical to monitor a dose of 50–100 ml from such a container and the patient is likely to receive more bicarbonate than he needs. Too much bicarbonate promotes both alkalosis and sodium overload and should be avoided. If the period of arrest is prolonged beyond 5 minutes, further bicarbonate will be required. It is not easy to assess additional requirements but an approximate guide is

$$\text{mEq bicarbonate} = \frac{\text{patient's weight in Kg} \times \text{period of arrest in minutes}}{10}$$

Defibrillation may be unsuccessful even after correction of acidosis. Coarse fibrillation is more responsive to defibrillation than the fine variety and prior injection of an anti-dysrhythmic drug may prove effective. A fine fibrillatory waveform may be rendered more coarse by giving 10 ml of 1 in 10,000 adrenaline intravenously.

Unfortunately, although it is nearly always possible to defibrillate the heart, effective myocardial contraction does not always accompany successful defibrillation. Failure to achieve palpable peripheral pulses from co-ordinated rhythm after 5–10 minutes is ominous.

Ventricular asystole

Complete absence of myocardial activity may be due to severe metabolic disturbance or a conduction block, but it usually indicates massive heart damage and is almost always fatal. In those cases which are *not* associated with massive muscle damage, asystole may be *transient,* due to delay in the emergence of a reliable pacemaker, or it may be *permanent*, e.g. following bilateral bundle branch block and the failure of a subsidiary pacemaker to arise spontaneously. An effective heart beat can sometimes be restored in such cases by

a) sharp blows to the praecordium
b) an intravenous bolus injection of 10 ml of 10% calcium chloride
c) an intravenous infusion of isoprenaline (2.5 mg in 500 ml 5% dextrose)
d) as a desperate measure, an injection of 10 ml of 1 in 10,000 adrenaline directly into the left ventricle.

Prophylactic insertion of a demand pacemaker will prevent asystole resulting from *conduction block.* There is usually adequate warning from increasing degrees of block or extreme bradycardia, but in some cases, the onset of asystole may be abrupt. Routine measures for the treatment of cardiac arrest must be instituted if the measures outlined above fail to restore a spontaneous effective heart beat, pending the insertion of a pervenous pacing electrode. External pacing can be tried as a temporary measure but is not usually satisfactory. If the patient survives, artificial pacing will be

Cardiac Dysrhythmias

continued until no further evidence of heart block remains; insertion of a permanent pacemaker may prove to be necessary.

On the whole, the prevention of ventricular asystole is much less successful than the prevention of fibrillation. Basically, if asystole follows conduction block in an otherwise relatively undamaged heart, there is a reasonable chance of survival, which is the reason why some units like to insert artificial pacemakers prophylactically. If there is extensive muscle damage, the prognosis is poor, even if resuscitative measures are initially effective in restoring or providing electrical activity and a co-ordinated muscle response. Massive muscle damage is associated with a poor cardiac output which becomes more and more ineffectual. Transient improvement can often be obtained from calcium chloride and isoprenaline, but the badly damaged heart is quite incapable of doing its job as a pump and death is inevitable.

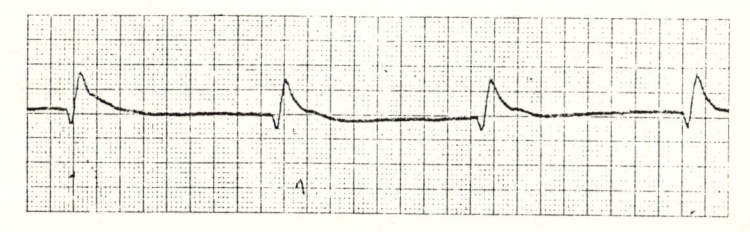

Fig. 14.23 The dying heart. There are no P waves, indicating atrial standstill. The QRS complexes are wide, with an irregular rate of about 40 per minute.

15

The Kidney

Greek — nephros, Latin — renalis, hence nephrectomy, nephrotic syndrome, nephritis, renal failure etc.

The basic unit of kidney function is the nephron. The nephron consists of the *glomerulus* with its renal tubes. The glomerulus (Latin — a ball) is a tuft of capillaries surrounded by a *glomerular capsule.* The capsule is the beginning of a succession of renal tubules which ultimately join collecting tubules and drain into the renal pelvis and the ureter. By folding the capillaries into a tuft and invaginating the thin walls of the flomerular capsule between the folds, a considerable surface area is made available for the filtration process which occurs in the glomerulus.

As the blood flows through the glomerular capillaries, a proportion of the *plasma* is filtered off from the capillaries into the capsule. Analysis of this

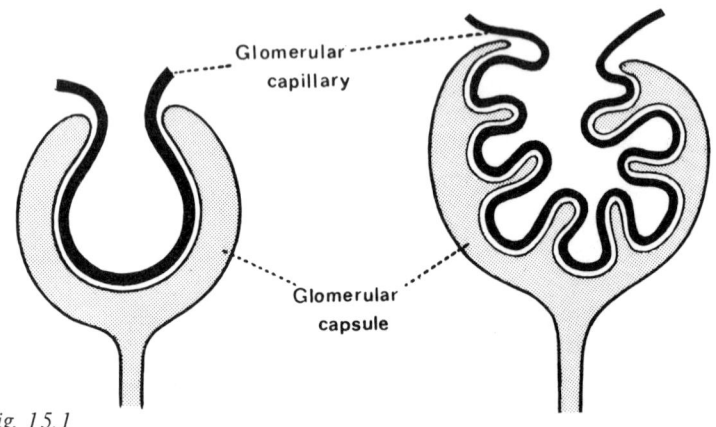

Fig. 15.1

filtrate shows that it contains the same concentrations of the ions and molecules present in the plasma, i.e. sodium, potassium, hydrogen, chloride and phosphate ions; urea, creatinine, glucose and the smaller protein molecules. Larger molecules and red blood cells do not normally pass through from the capillaries into the glomerular capsule.

The flow of blood through the kidney — the *renal blood flow* — is altered by various factors, e.g. exercise, anaesthesia, drugs, haemorrhage. The rate at which plasma is filtered into the glomerular capsule is called the *glomerular filtration rate*. When the renal blood flow deviates markedly from the normal range the rate of glomerular filtration is affected.

From the glomerulus, the filtrate passes into the *proximal convoluted tubule*. Here, all the glucose and most of the electrolytes are extracted from the filtrate by the tubule *cells*, together with the water required to maintain the concentration of those substances within the normal range in the blood. The extracted fluid is then reabsorbed into the blood via a network of capillaries which surrounds the renal tubules.

The smaller protein molecules which have passed through into the glomerular capsule are metabolised by the cells of the proximal tubule into amino-acids. Normally, about 50 grams — nearly one quarter of the total plasma protein — are metabolised daily in this way. These amino-acids are returned to the circulation via the tubular capillary network.

Approximately 20–24 ml remains of the original glomerular filtrate to be presented *per minute* to the *distal convoluted tubule* for further modification. In the distal tubule, sodium, hydrogen and potassium ions are reabsorbed or excreted as required, ammonia is formed, and water is reabsorbed or allowed to pass on according to the metabolic needs of the body.

The steroid hormone *aldosterone* promotes the excretion of unwanted hydrogen and potassium ions produced by metabolic activity. It also promotes the reabsorption of sodium ions to take their place. The kidneys normally excrete about 50 mEq of hydrogen ions every day but can increase the output to 600 mEq. The hydrogen ions are normally buffered — electrically neutralised — by *phosphate ions* which have not been reabsorbed in the proximal tubule. When hydrogen ion excretion occurs at a high rate for any length of time, the extra buffering capacity required is provided by *ammonia*. The ammonia, formed in the cells of the distal tubule, 'mops up' the hydrogen ions to produce ammonium ions.

Hydrogen ions are written	H^+
Mono-hydrogen phosphate ions	HPO_4''
Di-hydrogen phosphate ions	H_2PO_4'
Ammonium ions	NH_4^+
A molecule of ammonia	NH_3

The $^+$ and $'$ symbols indicate the number of positive and negative charges carried by the various ions.

$H^+ + HPO_4'' = H_2PO_4'$

$H^+ + NH_3 = NH_4^+$

The addition of one hydrogen ion (with one positive charge) to the mono-hydrogen phosphate ion (with two negative charges) produces the di-hydrogen phosphate ion, at the same time reducing the number of negative charges to one. Similarly, adding one hydrogen ion to the uncharged ammonia molecule creates the ammonium ion with one positive charge.

Substances in solution are called *solutes*. In the glomerular filtrate, the solutes in solution include the breakdown products of metabolism as well as glucose and electrolytes. The composition of the filtrate changes as the filtrate passes along the renal tubules. Furthermore, the kidney is able to produce variations both in the *concentration* and the *volume* of the fluid it ultimately produces as urine, according to the amount of solutes to be excreted and the water needs of the body. If there is an increase in the amount of solutes to be excreted, either the urine concentration must be increased also, or less water must be reabsorbed in order to carry the extra solutes in less concentrated urine. Of course, both these processes can and do occur simultaneously, in varying degrees appropriate to the requirements of the body at the time. However, an increase in urine volume due to an unusually heavy solute load is called an *osmotic diuresis*.

(crudely, osmos – to push)

osis – a process, therefore in combination, a pushing or inevitable process

diuresis – to make water)

Any water in the distal tubule which is not required for osmotic purposes (that is, for the carrying of solutes in solution) is either reabsorbed by the distal tubule and the collecting duct cells, or allowed to pass on to the renal pelvis to be excreted, according to the body's water requirements. The amount of this 'free' water is originally influenced by the quantity of the fluid filtered into the glomerular capsule (normally fairly constant) but the final adjustment of the urine volume is under the control of the antidiuretic hormone ADH. If the body requires water, ADH is secreted by the pituitary gland, and maximum reabsorption of the 'free' water occurs. If there is excess body water, e.g. due to generous drinking or vigorous intravenous fluid therapy, then ADH secretion is suppressed to allow unimpeded water excretion, or diuresis.

If water intake is restricted or if water cannot be absorbed normally via the alimentary tract, the distal tubules and collecting tubules will reabsorb water to the best of their ability, and a small quantity of concentrated urine will be passed. The minimum quantity of water required to excrete the normal daily solute load derived from metabolic processes is about 400 ml. If water intake or absorption is reduced to such an extent that this minimum output is greater than the intake of water, then a negative state of water balance exists and the patient starts to become dehydrated. Since solute concentration in the urine is already maximal, no further increase in solute excretion can occur and the concentration of solutes in the tubular fluid therefore rises. As a result, the solutes which should have been excreted pass back into the blood.

An increased concentration of urea in the blood, together with the other nitrogenous products of metabolism, is called *uraemia*; a rise in the concentration of hydrogen ions in the blood produces *acidaemia*. Other states may be described, e.g. hyperkalaemia (Kalium − Latin for potassium) and hypernatraemia (Natrium − Latin for sodium).

Renal Failure

There are two components to urine production − glomerular filtration and tubular function. Disordered renal function will depend on which of these components is affected. The renal tubules are very susceptible to ischaemia, for example, but have a remarkable capacity for regeneration. The glomeruli are less susceptible to ischaemic damage but if necrosis occurs as a result of infection or prolonged ischaemia, they are not capable of regeneration.

Renal failure may be acute or chronic.

Acute renal failure is by definition a condition in which the urine volume falls below the minimum necessary for the excretion of the solute load. This does not necessarily mean that the patient becomes obliguric, since the solute load may have increased, e.g. in burns cases. Failure of renal function is therefore not necessarily associated with oliguria or anuria. Chronic renal disease is often associated with a normal or excessive urine volume and the disorder may be one of quality rather than quantity. An adequate urine volume does not by itself indicate adequate urine function, which is why simple urine testing should be carried out on every patient.

The normal range of urine output varies from 600−1500 ml per day. A reduction in urine volume below 600 ml per day should be regarded as *oliguria*. *Anuria* means no urine and should be restricted to this situation.

Common Causes of Oliguria

Oliguria is not uncommon in Intensive Care patients. Many of them have indwelling *catheters* in the bladder and the flow of urine along them can become obstructed in various ways.

a) clots of blood or epithelial debris
b) kinking of the tubing, or obliteration of its lumen by external pressure
c) the valves of collecting bags may fail to work properly so that urine cannot siphon into the bag

Retention of urine is likely in the patient with prostatic hypertrophy or in the unconscious patient but in both cases, overflow of urine usually occurs eventually. Such patients should be catheterised initially to prevent this or relieve the condition should it arise. *Obstruction* to the flow of urine may follow trauma or surgery to the ureter, bladder or kidney, but this damage should be suspected from the history and the patient must be carefully observed for this development.

Most frequently, oliguria is the result of an *inadequate fluid intake* for the particular circumstances. Careful assessment of fluid balance is very important in any patient with an abnormal loss. Relatively small variations in fluid balance can, over two or three days, produce a deficit which may proceed unnoticed until revealed by oliguria.

Another common cause of oliguria is *inadequate perfusion* of the kidney. Episodes of hypotension in Intensive Care patients are not unusual and there may have been hypotensive periods prior to admission or during surgery. If the systolic blood pressure falls below 70 mmHg for more than a short period of time, glomerular filtration will often be reduced until the pressure has risen again. Longer periods of hypotension, or complete obstruction to renal blood flow for more than half an hour, will probably lead to renal tubular necrosis. Although the glomeruli are less susceptible to ischaemia than the renal tubules, any prolonged or gross impairment of renal blood flow may well lead to acute glomerular necrosis. This condition is likely to be irrecoverable since necrotic glomeruli cannot be replaced, but the prognosis does depend on the number of glomeruli involved. Kidneys seem to vary in their sensitivity to ischaemia however, and oliguria may develop unexpectedly in some patients and fail to do so in others who might have been thought vulnerable.

Body water and electrolytes

The amount of water in the body is related to the number of particles — ions and molecules — present in the various fluid compartments. This is because the *concentrations* of many of the ions and molecules are maintained by active metabolic processes within a certain range. The concentration of a solution is a measure of the amount of a substance present in the solution. If the balance between the intake and output of these particles is upset for any reason, their concentrations in the blood, and therefore in the extracellular fluid compartment generally, will be altered and the body will take steps to restore the situation to normal to the best of its ability. The sodium ion is the predominant positive ion in the extracellular fluid, so that a reduction in sodium intake, or an excessive loss, is likely to produce a marked effect.

Inadequate *salt* intake (or excessive salt loss without adequate replacement) leads to a reduction in the extracellular fluid sodium. In order to maintain the normal concentration of sodium, the kidney reabsorbs as much sodium, and excretes as much water, as it can. At the same time, the excessive amount of water in the extracellular fluid — excessive because the sodium content is reduced — is redistributed into the intracellular fluid compartment; more water is removed from the interstitial fluid component of the extracellular fluid than from the blood component owing to the presence of the plasma proteins, which tend to retain water in the blood. There is none the less an early fall in blood volume, causing haemoconcentration. Initially, sodium and chloride levels in the *blood* remain within normal limits, falling only when depletion is severe. Urine volume likewise remains normal until circulatory changes brought about by the fall in blood volume and haemoconcentration begin to affect the kidney. The patient suffers from lassitude and apathy; there is usually nausea, vomiting and intestinal ileus, which lead to further salt loss and aggravate the situation. Ultimately, vasoconstriction and circulatory failure occur, associated with obvious dessication of the skin, collapsed veins and a low ocular tension.

An inadequate *water* intake leads to a rise in the sodium and chloride concentrations in the extracellular fluid, i.e. there is a rise in extracellular fluid *osmolarity*. Osmolarity is another term for concentration. Its use indicates that the particles in solution can exert an osmotic effect. There is no physical barrier to the movement of ions between the intra- and extracellular fluids — but metabolic activity creates one. The rise in extracellular fluid osmolarity causes water to be redistributed from the intracellular fluid osmolarity causes water to be redistributed from the intracellular fluid into the extracellular fluid in an attempt to restore its osmolarity. As a result, that of the intracellular fluid rises. There is a lag in the process however and it is never fully complete, so that the blood sodium and chloride levels remain higher than normal, and the blood volume remains slightly reduced. The patient is thirsty, there is loss of skin elasticity, oliguria, and a high urine specific gravity due to maximum conservation of water.

The post-operative patient treated with an adequate fluid intake but inadequate salt is unlikely to come to any great harm however because

    a) the period of restricted oral intake is seldom prolonged

b) the kidneys can combat salt deficiency better than they can combat water deficiency
c) sodium in the bones forms a reserve which is usually adequate to cope with the period of intravenous therapy.

If however the post-operative period of intravenous therapy is associated with abnormal *losses* of salt and water, e.g.

alimentary secretions, fistulae, diarrhoea and vomiting, excessive intestinal aspirations

and unbalanced infusion therapy is provided or given for a long period, then not only can the salt depletion become severe but water depletion is also likely to occur. The effects on the patient will depend on the relative imbalance of the two conditions. The body will try to maintain the osmolarity of the extracellular fluid compartment — the concentration of *all* the solutes in the extracellular fluid — at all costs. Since the sodium ion is the predominant positive ion in the extracellular fluid, variation in its concentration produced by inadequate intake must affect the total extracellular fluid osmolarity. The response of the body to inadequate water and salt intake will thus depend not only on the relative imbalance of the intake but also on the presence of abnormal losses and any other effects due to abnormal pathology.

The management of oliguria

When a patient becomes oliguric, the nurse should first check that any catheter and its tubing is patent. Sometimes, merely detaching the collecting bag results in an immediate flow of a large quantity of urine that has been dammed back by a faulty valve in the bag. Clots and debris may be dislodged by flushing the catheter but they are frequently drawn back into it to block it once again, and a free flow may only be established after a thorough bladder wash-out.

Catheterisation is required both to exclude bladder neck obstruction and to enable the rate of urine production to be recorded. The patient should be carefully assessed for the presence or absence of thirst and abnormal elasticity of the skin. A dry tongue is not a helpful sign — the patient may be a mouth breather or keep his mouth open for much of the time. The fluid intake and output for the previous few days should be checked carefully with particular reference to abnormal losses, e.g. drains, fever, sweating, rapid respiration, vomiting, diarrhoea etc. All urine must be kept as 24-hour specimens; it will be examined for specific gravity, casts and red cells, electrolytes and urea content, and osmolarity (the concentration of all the solutes in the urine, measured in milliosmoles per litre). Incidentally, solute concentration can also be measured in terms of the *weight* of the fluid concerned as well as its volume, i.e. milliosmoles per kilogram instead of milliosmoles per litre; in this case, the term *osmolality* is used to describe the osmotic effects of the solutes in the fluid.

Renal damage is more likely to be responsible for oliguria if

1) there has been a recorded episode of hypotension or a low cardiac output
2) the specific gravity of the urine is less than 1010
3) there are casts and red blood cells in the urine
4) the urinary urea concentration is less than 11 grams in 24 hours.

'*Dehydration*', i.e. water and salt depletion, is suggested by

1) a negative or inadequate fluid balance
2) low blood pressure
3) reduced skin elasticity
4) the absence of oedema.

A urine specific gravity greater than 1010 may indicate inadequate fluid intake — unless there is some reason for the presence of excess solutes in the urine, e.g. dextrose or haemoglobin after cardio-pulmonary by-pass.

A urinary urea concentration of more than 11 grams in 24 hours suggests, but does not prove, that the cause of the oliguria is inadequate fluid intake — it only indicates satisfactory tubular function.

The following regime helps to assess the situation.

1) A Central Venous Pressure line is set up if one is not already present.
2) If the Central Venous pressure is low, Normal saline is given intravenously until pressure is at, or slightly above, the upper limit of normal.
3) 100 ml of 20% Mannitol is then given. Frusemide 250–1000 mg is often administered as well, particularly if there is any doubt as to the ability of the myocardium to cope with the temporary increase in circulating blood volume.

> If oliguria is due to pre-renal causes, the urine flow rate should increase to 1 ml/minute. If this flow rate does not occur, the cause of the oliguria is *probably* not pre-renal.

If the oliguria persists, then acute renal failure may be assumed to be present and restriction of fluid, food and salt intake must be instituted prior to starting renal dialysis, and any further investigations.

Fluid intake is restricted to 250 ml per square metre of surface area (on average, about 400 ml) per 24 hours *in addition* to the fluid output during the previous 24 hours. This includes vomit, faeces, urine, fluid loss from wounds etc.

A high carbohydrate diet is given in order to minimise protein breakdown, thereby delaying the progress of uraemia, e.g. Hycal (Beecham) which provides 240 calories per 100 ml, and a mixture created at the Royal Free

Hospital which provides 408 calories per 100 ml (this mixture has 5 grams of protein per 100 ml). Both possess minimal electrolyte concentration.

All drug dosages must be examined and reduced where necessary in order to prevent their concentrations in the blood rising to toxic levels, e.g. digitalis. Tetracyclines are contraindicated.

The use of ion exchange resins may be necessary in order to reduce plasma potassium levels. These remove potassium ions from the body, replacing them with sodium or calcium ions according to the resin used.

Dialysis

Greek   dia – through or across
             lysis – to lose or loosen

The walls of the glomerular capillaries and the glomerular capsule constitute a filter or *semi-permeable membrane*. The peritoneum can function in the same way, as can an artificial substance such as a sheet of cellophane – but as both these structures are considerably thicker than the layers of cells involved in filtration in the glomeruli, and as the surface area available for filtration in the kidney is estimated to be as much as one square metre, the filtration process naturally takes longer than in the kidney. Moreover, dialysis can only replace the filtration component of kidney function – it cannot provide the sensitive tubular component of selective reabsorption and secretion.

The principle of the method is to provide a concentration gradient across a semi-permeable membrane so that the tendency of ions and molecules to achieve an equal concentration on both sides of the membrane – a basic law of chemistry – induces them to pass from one fluid to another. Where a concentration gradient exists, the movement of ions and molecules from the fluid of higher concentration is greater than in the reverse direction. If the process were to be allowed to continue until the number of ions and molecules were equal on both sides of the semi-permeable membrane, then equilibrium would be achieved and at this point, the rate at which the particles pass in one direction is equal to their rate of passage in the other direction. Another basic law – ions and molecules are in constant motion so that even in a state of equilibrium, the particles continue to move about. In other words, equilibrium is a dynamic state, not a static one.

The movement of particles across a membrane in this way is called *diffusion*. The rate of diffusion decreases considerably as the concentration gradient is reduced, so that in dialysis, a more rapid and effective 'clearance' of unwanted substances from the blood is achieved if a reasonable concentration gradient is maintained. This is done by frequent changing of the dialysing fluid.

In peritoneal dialysis, 1–2 litres of the dialysing solution warmed to 37°C are run into the peritoneal cavity under the influence of gravity, like an intravenous infusion. Some units allow the fluid to remain there for 10–20 minutes before draining it off again into a collecting bag; some keep the fluid in the peritoneal cavity for a longer period, others use no 'dwell' time at all. Usually, about 30–60 minutes is allowed for the whole cycle, depending on the volume of fluid used. The giving set has two Y connections incorporated into it. The top one allows two dialysate bags to be

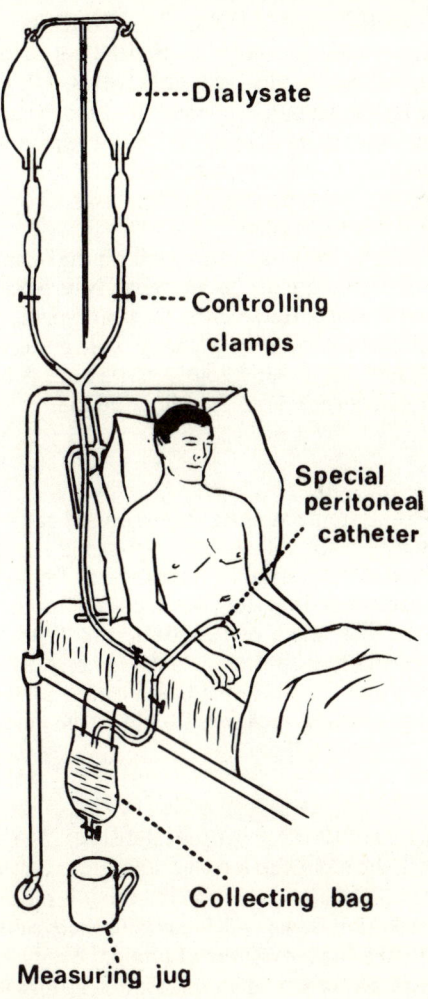

Fig. 15.2 Peritoneal dialysis.

connected at the same time, so that empty bags may be changed without interrupting the cycle; the lower one directs the dialysate into either the peritoneal cavity or the collecting bag.

The volumes passing in and out of the peritoneal cavity must be recorded at every cycle, because occasionally some of the dialysate can be retained in cavities formed by peritoneal folds. The effects of such loculation (Latin loculus — one of a number of small cavities) can often be overcome by re-positioning the catheter, or re-inserting it if necessary. The volumes of dialysate in and out must balance over 24 hours, otherwise the patient is in danger of becoming overloaded with water. Note that the 'litre' bags of dialysate actually contain on average about 1040 ml so that an apparent negative dialysate balance results — in other words, a 'litre' is put in but more than a litre is drained out; remember that the 'balance' refers to the dialysing fluid, *not* the patient's body fluids. An apparent negative balance of 40 multiplied by the number of bags used in 24 hours may thus occur and be accounted for. This apart, the balance over 12 or 24 hours must be assessed for each individual patient.

Mechanical methods are available to perform the in and out cycles and these are used in specialised units, as are weigh beds to keep a check on the patient's water balance. However, in most instances, careful measurement and recording of the volumes exchanged are perfectly satisfactory in the Intensive Care Unit if meticulously carried out. Simple charts are necessary and should cover a 12 and 24 hour period.

Asepsis

The dialysate must be sterile as must be peritoneal catheter, tubing and connections. Samples of the effluent dialysate are taken daily and examined for bacterial and fungal contamination. Prophylactic antibiotics have no place in peritoneal dialysis, but appropriate antibiotics can be added to the dialysate if peritonitis occurs. Their administration requires care, particularly with those which are normally excreted in the urine unchanged, as toxic levels in the blood can be achieved very easily. Where possible, blood antibiotic levels should be measured frequently.

The dialysate

Two main types are available for peritoneal dialysis. The electrolyte concentrations of each are identical, but one solution is only slightly hypertonic compared with the blood whereas the other is more strongly so.

A *hypertonic* solution is one which contains more substances per unit volume of fluid than a similar volume of blood. Usually, only one substance is in excess — dextrose, for example. Dialysate solutions do not contain protein, so if the solutions are to be hypertonic compared with blood, some other substance must be added to increase the tonicity. Dextrose (glucose) is particularly suitable. It is a normal constituent of blood and as some will inevitably pass into the blood during dialysis, it will provide a source of energy and help to avoid the breakdown of protein.

The *concentration* of a solution is the amount of any substance, expressed in any convenient units, present in a unit of weight, or a unit of volume, of the solution. Familiar examples are mg per ml, grams per litre, gram per gram, mEq per litre and so on. Whatever the units, a relationship exists between the solute and the solvent; and for any given concentration, alteration of one must be followed by alteration of the other if the concentration is to be maintained. The intracellular and extracellular fluid contains many substances in solution in water. The concentration of some of these, such as sodium, hydrogen and potassium, is strictly controlled by active metabolic processes. *Ions* form a large proportion of the particles present in the body fluids and are mainly responsible for the actual *volume* of water in the body. The strict control of the concentrations of some of the ions, in particular sodium, influences the *distribution* of water within the body; they have an *osmotic* effect, due not to the presence of a semipermeable membrane but to actively-maintained concentrations in spite of the ability, in most cases, to pass freely across cell membranes. The total concentration of the particles in the various body fluids can therefore be expressed in terms of *osmolarity*, measured in milliosmoles per litre, and a comparison made between the osmolarity of the blood and that of the dialysates.

	Blood	Dialysate I	Dialysate II
Osmolarity in m.osmoles/litre	310–320	364.37	642.91
Dextrose in grams/litre	1.0–1.2	13.6	63.6

If acute renal failure has led to an excessive volume of water in the body, this water will be distributed throughout the intracellular and extracellular fluid spaces, thus minimising the effect. The strongly hypertonic solution is used for a proportion of the dialysing cycles in order to remove this excess water. Water removed from the blood is replaced by water from the interstitial fluid so that the normal blood volume is maintained. Redistribution of water from the intercellular space into the interstitial space can then occur. The result is a reduction in total body water.

If the strongly hypertonic solution is used too frequently, water may be removed from the circulating blood faster than it can be redistributed from the other fluid compartments and the blood volume will be reduced. For this reason, the patient must be observed closely for any signs of hypovolaemia during dialysis and the pulse and blood pressure recorded regularly, particularly if the strongly hypertonic solution is being used.

Furthermore, if water is removed rapidly from the extracellular fluid by the use of hypertonic dialysate, the concentration of sodium ions in the extracellular fluid will tend to rise, because the transfer of water back from the intracellular fluid does not occur as quickly as the water is removed. Sodium ions therefore tend to be excreted with the water until redistribution of water has occurred, in order to maintain the osmolarity of the extracellular fluid. This process is called 'solvent drag'. The hypertonic solution also causes considerable abdominal discomfort, so it is preferable to restrict fluid intake in patients undergoing peritoneal dialysis in order to avoid unnecessary use of the strong solution.

Electrolyte composition of the dialysates compared with the blood

	Blood	Dialysate I	Dialysate II
Sodium in mEq/l	137–149	140.4	140.4
Calcium mEq/l	4.2–5.4	3.6	3.6
Chloride mEq/l	97–107	100.8	100.8

The electrolyte concentrations of the dialysates are essentially those of the lower level of the normal range in the blood, so there is no danger of too rapid or excessive removal of electrolytes from the blood. Note that there are no potassium ions in the standard dialysate solutions. Patients in acute renal failure are more likely to be hyperkalaemic than hypokalaemic, and experience has shown that it is safer to dialyse without potassium ions until the blood concentrations are within the normal range, after which 4 mEq/l of potassium are added to the dialysate prior to running it into the peritoneal cavity.

Peritoneal dialysis can be maintained for several weeks provided that the greatest care is taken to maintain sterile precautions. In the majority of cases, renal function will be restored within 3–4 weeks. If there is evidence that dialysis will be necessary for a longer period, then haemodialysis should be considered.

Complications of peritoneal dialysis

1) Peritonitis
   Perforation of abdominal organs
   Displacement of the catheter
   Leakage of dialysis fluid
   Improper drainage
   Pain

2) Fluctuations in blood volume, and sodium and potassium ion concentration in the blood

   Hyperglycaemia

Advantages of peritoneal dialysis — No complicated apparatus is required. There is no need for blood to prime a machine nor heparin to prevent clotting. Most important of all, it does not require specially trained staff. It is however less efficient than haemodialysis, and although once the acute metabolic imbalance has been rectified by continuous exchanges the patient can be maintained by intermittent dialysis, this will probably be necessary every night as opposed to two or three times a week using haemodialysis.

Haemodialysis

Blood from the patient is passed through sterile tubing made from a substance which will act as a semi-permeable membrane, and the tubing is immersed in the dialysing solution.

Originally, blood was taken from the Inferior Vena Cava, cannulated via a cut-down on the femoral vein in the groin, and returned to the patient via another cannula placed in any suitable large peripheral vein.

This *veno-venous* method is rarely performed today. Sepsis is common as is vena caval thrombosis. The method is suitable only for short-term dialysis when peritoneal dialysis is not feasible and the patient is very ill, since it requires only two simple cut-down procedures.

Arterio-venous dialysis The development of plastic materials has made long-term dialysis in chronic renal disease a practical possibility. The method is used however for both chronic and acute renal disease. One cannula is inserted into a peripheral artery, another into a suitable neighbouring vein and the two are joined together by pieces of tubing, making an arterio-venous shunt. Various designs of cannulae or 'shunts' are available. One in common use is the Scribner shunt, named after the person who developed it. The plastic materials employed are Silastic and Teflon.

Any suitable vessels may be used, such as the radial artery in the forearm and the posterior tibial in the ankle, both of which have reasonably large veins near them. The life of an artificial shunt of this nature varies from a couple of months to several years. Potential problems are

a) dislodgement of the shunt with resulting haemorrhage
b) sepsis
c) clotting — arising from trauma to the intima of the vessel from the cannulae
                          infection

                          hypotension

The cannulae and tubing must be firmly fixed in order to prevent dislodgement and to minimise trauma to the vessels. Nurses should listen over the shunt with a stethescope for a bruit at least three times a day and observe it for separation of clotted blood. To facilitate this, the tube should be covered with a dressing which leaves a small segment visible to detect clotting. Never take the blood pressure in an arm containing a shunt, or

a

Shunt tubing

Skin

Vessel   **Cannula**   **Vessel**

b Looking from on top

Shunt tubing

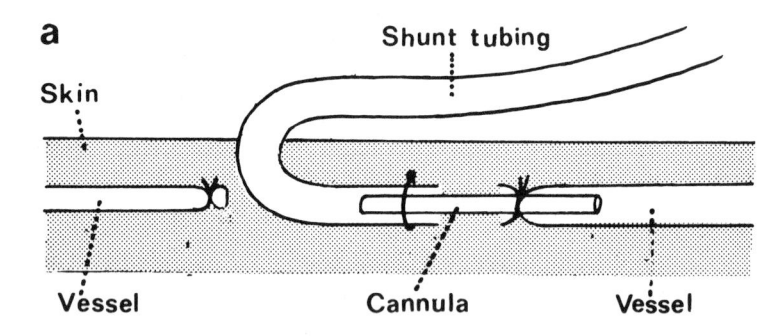

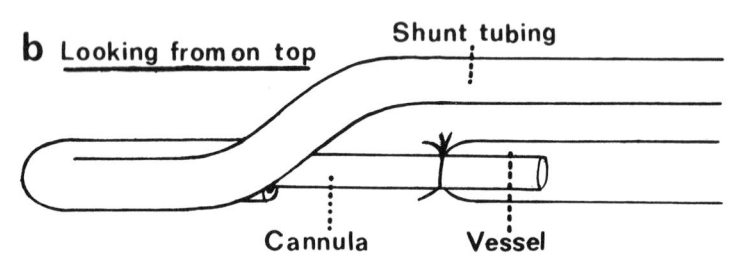

Cannula   **Vessel**

Fig. 15.3 The shunt tubing has 2 permanent curves incorporated into it. Diagram (a) illustrates the curve which brings the tubing out to lie on the surface of the skin. The second curve is a sideways one — a kink— which directs the tubing away from line of the cannula in the vessel, thus avoiding compression of the vessel by the tubing lying above it.

allow stasis to occur in the limb by placing the patient on his side, for example. Drugs must not be injected through the shunt under any circumstances because they may irritate the vessel walls and cause thrombosis, but shunts may be used for arterial blood sampling provided that a full aseptic technique is employed.

If clotting does occur, the connecting loop is disconnected and attempts are made to clear the cannulae by gentle irrigation with warm heparinised saline and by suction, using a syringe. Inserting a fine catheter up the cannulae and irrigating through the catheter will usually dislodge the clot.

Arterio-venous fistula

This method of access to the circulation has been developed for long-term dialysis in patients with *chronic* renal disease. An arterio-venous fistula is created surgically in the arm or leg. After a few weeks, the increased flow of blood through the fistula results in a considerable increase in the size of the veins draining the fistula. These veins are used for percutaneous puncture with large bore needles through which blood can be withdrawn and returned to the patient during dialysis. The method avoids some of the problems associated with external plastic shunts such as clotting and damage to the cannulated vessels. It is unlikely to be seen in the Intensive Care unit unless the patient has been admitted for other reasons.

The actual technique of haemodialysis will be far more easily understood by practical experience in the renal unit and I do not propose to discuss this.

16

Acute Respiratory Failure

Failure to draw oxygenated air into the lungs will lead to:

    hypoxia   — insufficient oxygen reaching the lungs

    hypercarbia   — a build-up of unexcreted carbon dioxide

and ultimately cardiac arrest.
This may occur as a result of

1) Absence of oxygen in the atmosphere — fume filled room, child with its head in a plastic bag.

2) Acute obstruction of the upper airway preventing breathing, in spite of adequate effort to do so.

    faciomaxillary injuries
burns, saliva, secretions, blood, vomit, foreign bodies, corrosive fluids, spasm of the glottis (as in the first $1\frac{1}{2}$ minutes of drowning) epiglottitis, quinsy, Ludwig's angina

3) Failure to ventilate adequately

    neuromuscular   cerebral trauma or depression, spinal injury, myasthenia, polyneuritis, tetanus
pulmonary   chronic bronchitis, asthma, pneumothorax
chest injuries

Acute Respiratory Failure

4) Failure to transport oxygen in the blood (hypoxaemia) — oedema of the lung, haemorrhage, denial of Haemoglobin (carbon monoxide poisoning, rupture of red cells in fresh water drowning)

In all cases, treatment involves attempting to obtain and maintain

> a clear airway
> adequate ventilation
> oxygenation

Always try to ensure that there is nothing obstructing the mouth or pharynx. Place a finger deep inside the mouth and sweep it round behind the tongue to remove vomit, food debris or foreign body. A foreign body producing acute airway obstruction may often be dislodged by a sharp blow on the back, particularly if the patient is a child and can be held upside down.

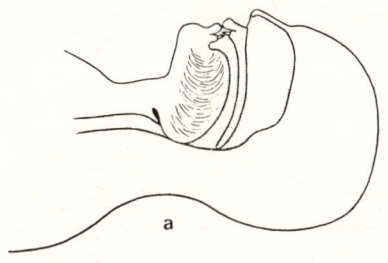

Fig. 16.1a The tongue has fallen back, obstructing the airway.

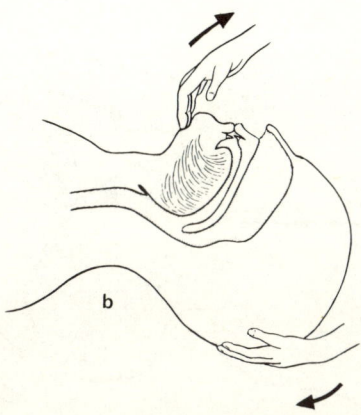

Fig. 16.1b 'Pulling up' the jaw, and extending the head on the neck will obtain a clear naso-pharyngeal airway in many cases.

Pull up (i.e. forward) the jaw to close the mouth, and extend the head fully — in most cases, this manoeuvre will prevent the tongue falling back in the pharynx and occluding the airway.

If the patient still fails to breathe in spite of a clear airway, the simplest and most effective means of inflating the lungs is *expired air ventilation*, using the *mouth-to-nose* method.

Take a few deep breaths first to ensure maximum oxygen concentration in your own lungs. Hold the jaw up with one hand, apply your mouth to the patient's nose (with your lips wide apart to avoid compressing the nostrils), and blow firmly, watching the patient's chest as you do so. The chest will rise provided there is no airway obstruction.

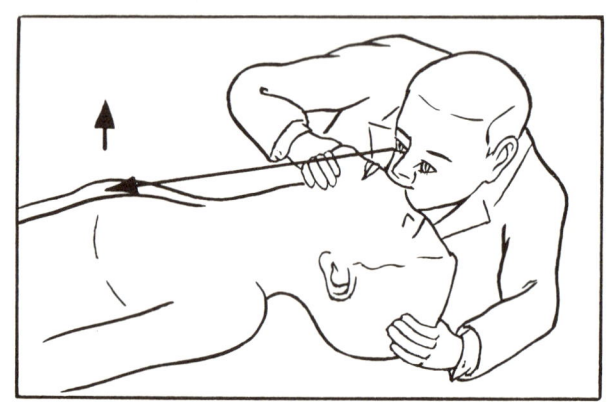

Fig. 16.2 Inflating the lungs, watching the chest rise at the same time.

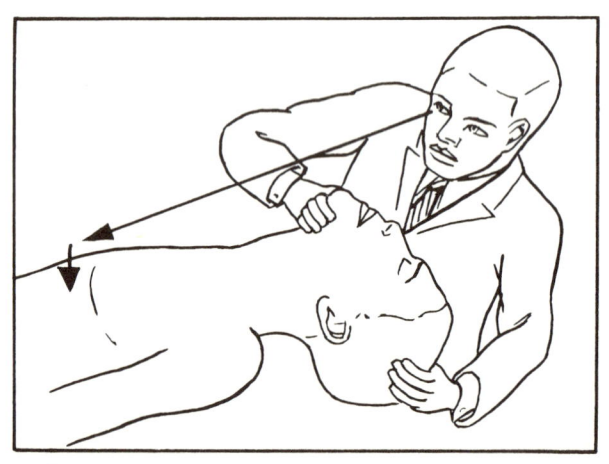

Fig. 16.3 Expiration — watching the chest wall fall as the lungs empty.

Acute Respiratory Failure

Brook airway

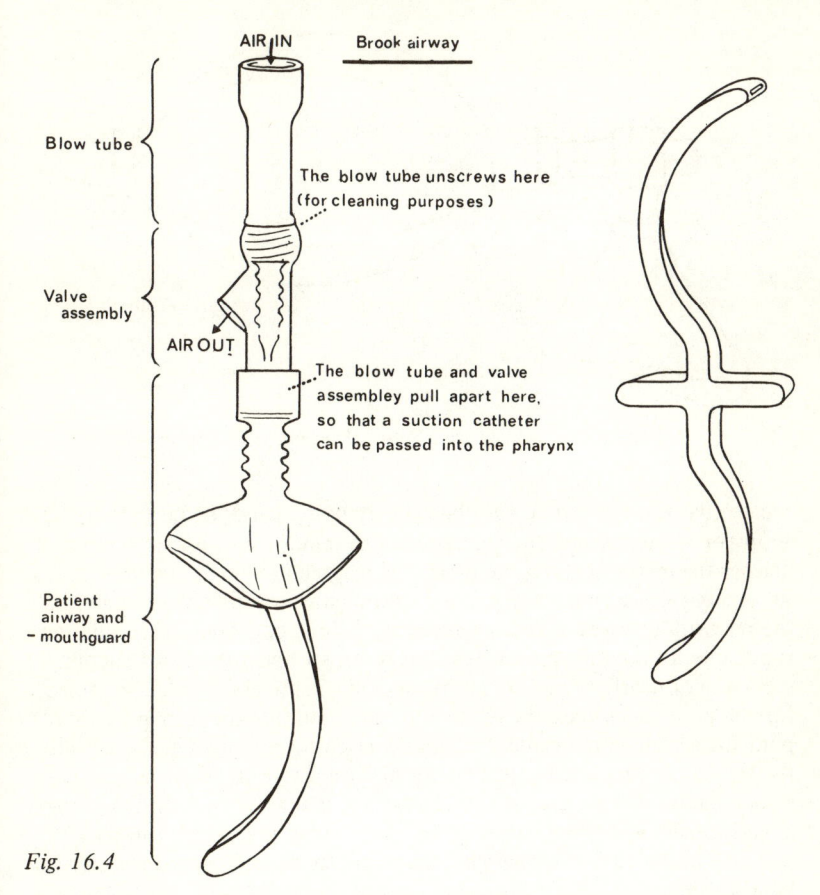

- Blow tube — AIR IN
- The blow tube unscrews here (for cleaning purposes)
- Valve assembly — AIR OUT
- The blow tube and valve assembley pull apart here, so that a suction catheter can be passed into the pharynx
- Patient airway and mouthguard

Fig. 16.4

Take your mouth from the patient's nose to allow the air to escape from the lungs through the nose, and watch the chest return to the resting position. Mouth-to-mouth ventilation may be necessary if there is any degree of nasal obstruction. The patient's nose is occluded by pinching with the fingers, while you blow into the mouth. With this method, it is difficult to get an airtight fit and the tongue is more likely to fall back and obstruct the airway since the mouth must be open, and furthermore, it is more difficult to watch the chest rise while blowing into the mouth.

The S-shaped airway and the Brook airway help to overcome these problems and in addition keep the resuscitator away from the patient's mouth.

In a hospital, a face mask, non-rebreathing valve and self-inflating bag or bellows are usually provided for emergency treatment.

If there is obstruction to the airway below the hypopharynx, or in the larynx or trachea, then simple measures to obtain a clear airway will be

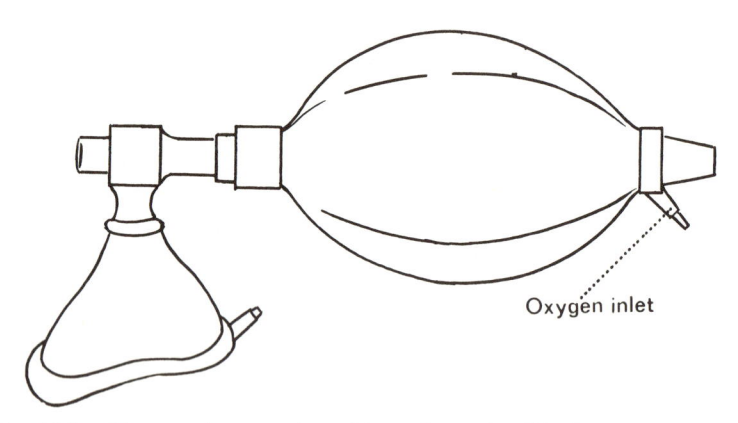

Fig. 16.5 Face mask, non-rebreathing valve and self-inflating bag.

ineffective and expired air ventilation may not expand the lungs. Laryngoscopy or bronchoscopy may be required to remove the obstruction, but neither the instruments or the personnel may be available. The indications for emergency laryngotomy or tracheotomy are fortunately very rare. In the majority of cases of acute ventilatory failure, endotracheal intubation is possible. In the rare cases where this is not so, and airway obstruction is complete or nearly so (severe glottic oedema, acute epiglottitis, impacted foreign body etc.), then the relatively simple but life-saving manoeuvre of plunging a wide-bore needle through the crico-thyroid membrane, or into the trachea, is much safer than emergency tracheotomy, especially in unskilled hands. The resistance to airflow is, of course, considerable but even a No 1 needle will allow a flow of 2–3 litres a minute, which can be lifesaving — provided further help arrives promptly so that other measures can be instituted.

There are various designs of tracheotome available for emergency tracheotomy. Most are simple to use — but it may be necessary to read the instructions first since, the indications for emergency tracheotomy being rare, the operator is most unlikely even to have handled the instrument. Under the circumstances, the procedure may well be complicated and even unsatisfactory.

The use of the resuscitator bag with a face mask.

Inflating the lungs with a face mask and bag under emergency conditions is *not* easy. Always inset an oral airway before attempting to inflate the lungs since the slightest obstruction to ventilation will result in some air passing into the stomach. A build-up of pressure, augmented by the effects of cardiac massage, if this is being carried out as well, is likely to lead to regurgitation. Some of this material will inevitably be 'blown' into the lungs and pulmonary complications added to the patient's problems.

You cannot hope to inflate the lungs using a face mask without a reasonably airtight fit. It is worth while practising holding a face mask correctly in the anaesthetic room or on the face of a sympathetic colleague.

The thumb and forefinger hold the mask against the patient's face; the other three fingers hook under the lower jaw. The main action is *apposition* of the thumb to the three fingers under the jaw — the thumb presses forwards and downwards while the three fingers under the jaw pull upwards and backwards. If the patient's neck is sweaty or greasy, the fingers will tend to slip. A piece of gauze under the fingers helps to provide a better grip.

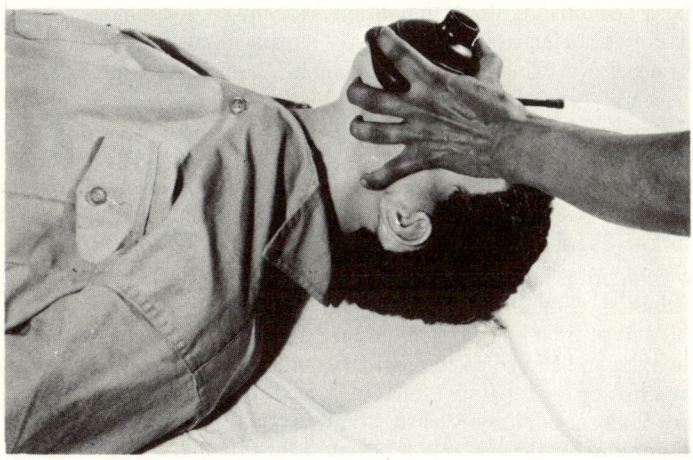

Fig. 16.6

If there is airway obstruction, it will be difficult to squeeze the bag and air will escape from underneath the mask. If you have not obtained an airtight fit, it will be easy to squeeze the bag and air will again escape from under the mask. In both cases there will be minimal or absent chest movement. If the chest does not rise and fall as you squeeze and release the bag, you are wasting your time. Check that the oral airway is correctly placed. Pull up the chin, replace the face mask and try again. If the patient is edentulous, you may need both hands to hold the mask onto the face, using the palms to 'gather up' the cheeks and force them against the sides of the mask. In this case, someone else will have to squeeze the bag. Sometimes, a bigger mask will solve the problem. Two hands will probably also be needed where the patient has a short, thick neck. In such cases, it is often very difficult to 'hook' the fingers under the jaws with one hand, particularly if your hands are small. The alternative of placing the ring and little fingers under the *angles* of the jaw, and lifting the whole lower jaw upwards and forwards may be the only way of maintaining the airway. Again, someone else will have to squeeze the bag.

A cuffed endotracheal tube should replace the oral airway and face mask if effective spontaneous ventilation is not resumed within a few minutes.

Subsequent treatment of acute respiratory failure

Once a cuffed tube has been passed through the mouth into the trachea and the cuff inflated, effective ventilation is assured in most cases and the danger of inhaling stomach contents is removed. If spontaneous ventilation is inadequate and is likely to remain so, mechanical ventilation will be necessary. While arrangements are being made for transfer to the Intensive Care or other special unit, the patient should be made comfortable and if conscious, reassured and sedated. There may be no special facilities available and a side room or part of a general ward will have to be used instead. Manual ventilation will be continued until the mechanical ventilator is ready. It is important not to over-ventilate the patient when inflating the lungs by hand. Reducing the carbon dioxide tension of the blood below 25 mmHg through over-ventilation can induce cardiac irregularities and reduce cerebral blood flow. Excessive ventilation can also reduce the cardiac output by inhibiting the venous return to the heart. Keep a finger on the pulse and an eye on the patient's colour until adequate supervision and monitoring facilities are available. A mechanical sucker must be available for tracheal or pharyngeal suction if necessary and 100% oxygen should be administered if there is any doubt as to the effectiveness of the patient's oxygenation. The flow rate necessary will vary according to the resuscitator bag in use and should be reduced if the bag shows a tendency to distend, and becomes difficult to squeeze.

Further treatment such as bronchial lavage, the appropriate antidote for poisons or corrosive fluids, the use of muscle relaxants to overcome spasm and the insertion of chest drains to relieve a tension pneumothorax may be required.

17

Cardiac Arrest Outside Specialised Treatment Areas

Although cardiac arrest is frequently a complication of myocardial disease, it can occur unexpectedly in young or middle-aged patients who might otherwise expect to enjoy a reasonable span of life. With this in mind, no effort should be spared to ensure successful resuscitation even if there are many disappointments.

Speed and teamwork are essential factors in the treatment of this emergency. Cerebral necrosis occurs within 2–4 minutes after circulatory arrest, so the fact that the heart has stopped beating must be recognised as soon as possible and the emergency drill immediately set in motion. Although treatment should be started by the nursing staff, extra help is necessary and must be summoned urgently. A special telephone number should be retained for this purpose only and the doctors on call must carry a special emergency bleep. An occasional visit to the staff manning the telephone exchange can pay dividends as their continued understanding and co-operation is of vital importance.

Equipment

Emergency boxes should ideally be provided in every ward, department or treatment area. If this is not possible, every ward and department should at least be equipped with a Brook airway so that effective resuscitation can be started by the nursing staff.

Mouth-to-nose or mouth-to-mouth ventilation can be life-saving in the street or railway station, but it should not be necessary to ask nurses to do this on the wards. The rest of the equipment can be brought to the patient by the doctors on call, one box serving the whole hospital apart from special

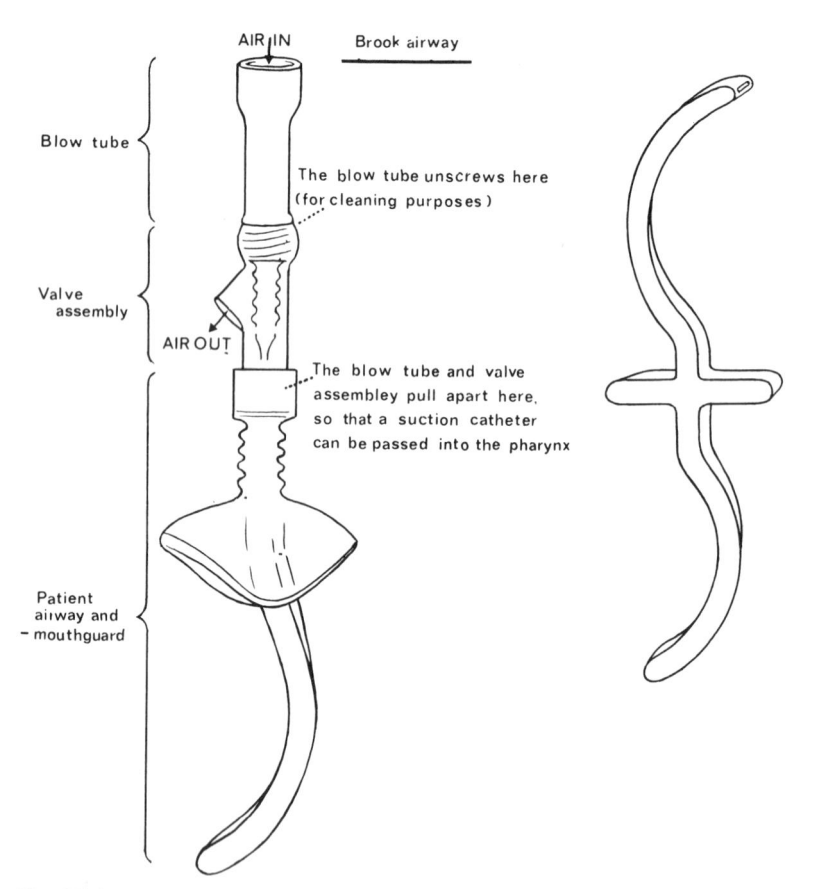

Fig. 17.1

areas such as casualty or the Intensive Care unit. A mechanical sucker should in any case be available on every ward. Even if expense is a bar to providing emergency boxes for every ward, it should be possible to provide all wards with a stout wooden board about 3′6″ by 2′6″ to fit across the bed. External cardiac massage performed on a patient in the standard hospital bed merely bounces the patient up and down; effective compression of the heart between the anterior chest wall and the vertebral column requires firm support for the body, and inserting a board under the patient is less traumatic for both patient and nurses than pulling the patient out of bed onto the floor. *Contents of emergency boxes* will vary from one hospital to another but the basic equipment is likely to include the following:

Laryngoscope, with long blade. This blade can be used satisfactorily for all ages, even neonates, but appropriate paediatric equipment should be provided in the obstetric and paediatric wards.

Plastic cuffed endotracheal tubes size 9, 8, 5, cut to appropriate length and with their connectors in place. They should be stored as 'clean' equipment in plastic bags.

Catheter mount

Self-inflating resuscitator bag, with non-return valve

Mitchell puffer for inflating the cuff of the endotracheal tube — the pilot tube will have its own stopper.

Oral airways — sizes 1, 2, 3.

Face masks — large, medium and small.

Brooke airway, through which the lungs may be inflated as a first aid measure by the single-handed resuscitator

1" bandage for tying-in the endotracheal tube

Intravenous cannulae, needles, syringes, infusion sets, adhesive strapping, gauze or other swabs,

Drugs — Adrenaline (10 ml of 1 in 10,000) Calcium chloride (10 ml of 10%) Lignocaine (20 ml of 1%) Isoprenaline (2.5 mg in 1 ml)

Oscilloscopes and defibrillators

The Intensive Care unit, Coronary Care unit, resuscitation area in Casualty etc. will have their own defibrillator, monitoring facilities and other specialised equipment, but it is not feasible to provide such facilities for the rest of the hospital. If only one defibrillator is available for the general wards, it may well be kept in the operating theatre suite; otherwise, a defibrillator and oscilloscope should be made available on a geographical basis and placed strategically to serve a group of wards or departments. The transport of equipment around the hospital is often a problem; nurses frequently find themselves fetching special equipment, usually because they do know where it is, what to look for or how to find it. In principle, this is to be depreciated, since a nurses place is at the bedside. A hospital porter would make a valuable member of the emergency team in this respect, but difficulties may arise over lack of continuity, and availability.

The equipment provided throughout the hospitals of the country varies considerably. There are still AC defibrillators in use and it is not unusual to find that the hospital ECG machine must be used for diagnostic and monitoring purposes during cardiac arrest. The Cardiac Recorders DC defibrillator, with or without its oscilloscope in a purpose built trolley, is found in many hospitals. It has the disadvantage that it is not portable in the strict sense of the word, and is mains operated. Equipment used in areas outside special units should really be portable and battery-operated. Portable combined defibrillator-oscilloscopes are now available, including models which use the defibrillator paddles to receive the ECG signals; these are particularly convenient for emergency use.

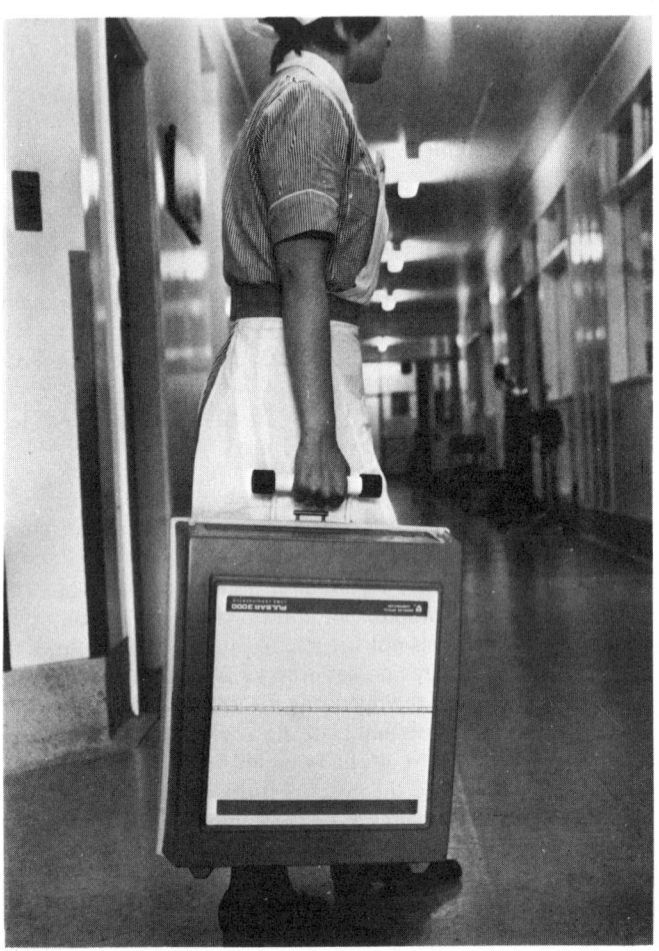

Fig. 17.2 A portable defibrillator.

The team available on the emergency bleep should include an anaesthetist since cardiac arrest outside special areas is usually unexpected and delay in starting resuscitation is almost inevitable. Artificial ventilation and cardiac massage are nearly always necessary and although ventilation must be started immediately with a Brook airway, or a face mask and Ambu bag, these methods provide no safeguard against aspiration of gastric contents, and the patient should be intubated as soon as possible in order to provide safe and efficient ventilation.

Successful resuscitation depends not only upon the speed with which resuscitation is started but also on whether the heart stops in ventricular fibrillation or asystole. The presence of *fibrillation* implies that the heart muscle fibres are at least capable of contracting, if only their activity can be properly co-ordinated. *Asystole* usually follows massive necrosis of the anterior wall and septum of the heart, with damage to both bundle branches; if a subsidiary pacemaker does arise, it will be a ventricular one, relatively slow and unreliable. Artificial pacing is therefore essential — but the survival rate is low. Asystole following sinus bradycardia or bundle branch block *without* massive muscle damage is a different matter. In such cases, the heart can often be 'paced' by sharp blows to the praecordium and if this manoeuvre produces palpable peripheral pulses, the method is preferable to external cardiac massage. If the heart can be paced in this way, an effective spontaneous heart beat may often be restored by a bolus dose of 10 ml of 10% Calcium chloride intravenously, or by an infusion of isoprenaline. The restoration of a spontaneous and effective cardiac output following such treatment indicates that a reliable subsidiary pacemaker has emerged in the atrium or atrio-ventricular node. Asystole following complete heart block is usually only temporary, and may not require pacing.

Successful *defibrillation* is greatly enhanced by the time interval between the onset of arrest and the administration of a DC shock. It is now generally agreed that experience and training in the safe use of the DC defibrillator should be given to nurses in charge of a Coronary Care or other special unit. This means that patients in such units can be defibrillated within 30 seconds of their arrest and their chances of successful resuscitation enormously enhanced. In these circumstances, cardiac massage and artificial ventilation are often unnecessary, unless palpable peripheral pulses do not accompany the restoration of a spontaneous co-ordinated contraction. If there are no palpable peripheral pulses one minute after the onset of fibrillation, during which a maximum of two shocks have been given in rapid succession followed by four or five sharp blows to the praecordium to stimulate the heart into activity, then external cardiac massage and artificial ventilation must be started without delay.

The Treatment of Cardiac arrest outside specialised areas

Cardiac arrest in these circumstances is usually always unexpected. The nurse may see the patient collapse or be called to the bedside by another patient. Although one may expect and hope that a nurse will not be on her own in such an emergency, she should nevertheless be quite clear in her mind what she has to do and the order in which to do it if such a situation arises.

Cardiac arrest is associated with the following:

1) sudden and unexpected loss of consciousness or 'collapse'. It is possible that the patient may have fainted, but in that case, there should be a palpable peripheral pulse, albeit a slow one, and the patient remains breathing regularly.
2) the absence of peripheral pulses − radial, femoral, carotid.
3) cyanosis or pallor − this will be influenced by the patient's complexion and the haemoglobin concentration.
4) absent or irregular gasping respiration.
5) dilatation of the pupils − not necessarily maximal but at least half-dilated.

If a patient suddenly collapses, the nurse must immediately feel for a peripheral pulse − which pulse depends on factors such as obesity and the presence of intravenous infusions, dressings etc. It can be difficult, for instance, to locate the carotid pulse in a fat patient with a thick short neck. If there is any doubt, it is better to assume that there is no pulse rather than waste valuable time making a prolonged check. The nurse should immediately give 3 or 4 sharp blows to the praecordium since there is a small chance of restoring co-ordinated contraction if the heart is in asytole following bundle branch block without massive myocardial damage. If no pulses are palpable following this manoeuvre, the nurse must immediately summon the cardiac arrest team. A special telephone number and adequate briefing of the staff of the telephone exchange should ensure minimum delay; the nurse should only have to say 'cardiac arrest, X ward' for her summons for help to be effective. The emergency box and bed board should be kept in the most convenient and accessible place − ideally by the telephone, since this is the first place to which a nurse will have to go before starting to treat the emergency. If two nurses are available, one will go to the telephone and bring the box and board with her on her return, while her colleague removes any pillows and gets the patient flat in bed. The patient is rolled onto his side so that the board can be pushed as far across the bed as possible and the patient is then rolled back onto the board. One of the nurses will start external cardiac massage while her colleague takes an oral airway, face mask and Ambu bag from the box. As soon as she is ready to inflate the lungs, external cardiac massage should be interrupted so that the lungs may be inflated 2 or 3 times. The chest is then compressed 4 or 5 times, the lungs are inflated once, the chest is compressed 4 or 5 times and this cycle of cardiac compression and lung inflation is continued until help arrives. If a supply of oxygen is close to hand, a flow rate of 2 litres per minute should be connected to the Ambu bag.

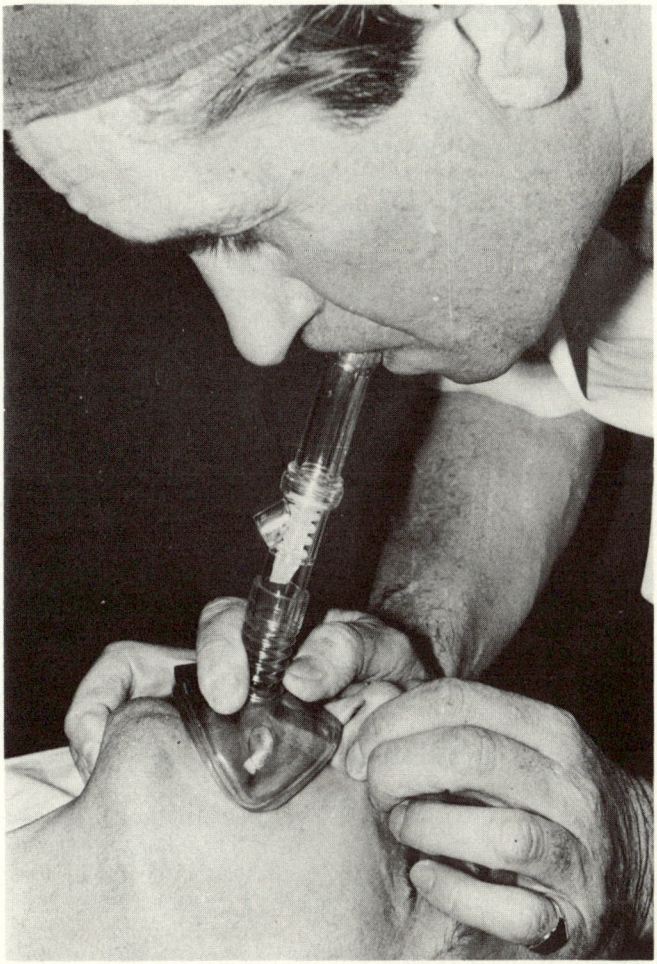

Fig. 17.3

The nurse on her own must do all this herself. Having telephoned for help, she must bring the box and board to the patient, remove any pillows and lie the patient flat. Probably the easiest way of placing the board under the patient will be to rest the board against the bed-head, pull the patient over towards her so that his body is propped against her, reach the board with both hands and place it flat on the bed with its proximal edge as close to the patient's body as possible and then push the patient over onto his back on the board.

Taking the Brook airway from the box, she should insert it in the patient's mouth, pull up the jaw and inflate the lungs twice. She should then compress the chest 10 or 12 times before repositioning the Brook airway and inflating the lungs twice again. External cardiac massage and artificial ventilation is continued in this fashion until help arrives.

As soon as medical help arrives, the patient is intubated and another person should take over cardiac massage. It is very important to maintain a regular rota for massage because one person cannot usually maintain efficient massage for longer than 2 or 3 minutes, particularly if they are doing it standing beside a patient on a bed. As soon as the patient is intubated, one of the nurses can take over ventilation again while an intravenous infusion is set up and 50–100 mEq of sodium bicarbonate is run in as fast as possible. The patient's legs should be raised in order to increase the return of blood to the heart and reduce the capacity of the circulation. If oxygen has not already been administered, it should be started immediately. The flow rate should be adjusted so that the inflating bag does not tend to over-distend or 'blow up' — a rate of 2–4 litres per minute is usually adequate.

It is worthwhile giving an immediate DC shock as soon as the defibrillator arrives without waiting to see whether the heart is fibrillating or not. The chances of successful defibrillation are reduced the longer a DC shock is delayed. If the heart is in asytole, a DC shock is ineffective but harmless. Procedure will vary slightly according to the type of equipment available. Some of the portable, battery-operated defibrillators now available have a rapid charging time of about 12 seconds; some models use the defibrillator paddles to receive the ECG signals so that an immediate diagnosis can be obtained. The mains-operated Cardiac Recorders defibrillator is commonly used with an oscilloscope which employs standard metal plates and limb leads so these must be strapped in place before an ECG is obtained. The maximum charge of 400 joules should be used when the heart has been fibrillating for more than 30 seconds. No-one, including the operator, should be touching the patient or the bed when the shock is delivered.

Effective contact between the paddles and the patient's skin is ensured by using the special jelly provided. Only enough jelly should be used to cover the area of skin in contact with the paddles. The blob of jelly is squeezed onto the skin where the paddles are to be placed; the paddles are then pressed firmly over the blobs and rotated a couple of times in order to spread out the jelly underneath them. If too much jelly is used, it is liable to spread over a wide area of skin and it is then possible for the

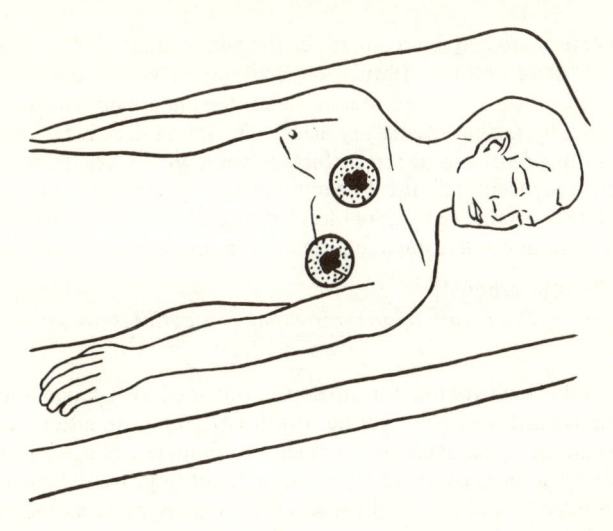

Fig. 17.4 Blobs of electrode jelly are placed
1) on the praecordium, i.e. over the heart
2) well to the left side of the chest. The actual position is not important.

two paddle areas to be linked by a continuous smear of jelly. This is equivalent to an electrical 'short circuit' and when a shock is given, the current may well arc from one paddle to another. Not only will defibrillation be ineffective, but the patient is likely to sustain quite severe burns to the skin in contact with the paddles. Too much jelly can also lead to it getting onto the upper surfaces of the paddles and onto the hands of the operators which could be dangerous.

Only the special electrode jelly should be used. Under no circumstances should KY jelly be used. It has no conducting properties — which are essential — and therefore resists the flow of current instead of assisting it.

Successful defibrillation is followed by a short period of asystole. QRS complexes may appear spontaneously after a few seconds but if they do not appear within 5 seconds, a succession of sharp blows to the chest will usually stimulate the heart into activity. The appearance of QRS complexes does not mean that external cardiac massage is no longer necessary; *effective* spontaneous contraction may well lag behind the restoration of normal electrical activity and cardiac massage is essential until co-ordinated rhythm is accompanied by a palpable pulse.

If defibrillation is unsuccessful or the heart cannot be stimulated into co-ordinated activity by a few blows to the chest, artificial ventilation and external cardiac massage must be resumed without delay. Further doses of sodium bicarbonate may be required, or the administration of an antidysrhythmic drug, before defibrillation is attempted once more.

Sodium bicarbonate is used to counteract the metabolic acidosis which builds up rapidly during circulatory arrest. The initial dose is 50–100 mEq but for prolonged periods of arrest, further doses will be necessary. It is difficult to judge accurately the dose required if only because it is not usually practical to take arterial samples of blood during a period of cardiac arrest. An approximate guide to additional requirements is provided by the formula

$$\text{mEq sodium bicarbonate} = \frac{\text{period of arrest in minutes} \times \text{patients' weight in kgm}}{10}$$

A conveniently small volume for infusion is provided by a concentration of 8.4% which is equal to 1 mEq per ml. Bottles of 100 ml should be available for use in cardiac arrest because too much bicarbonate will produce an alkalosis and a sodium overload. Alkalosis will not improve the chances of defibrillation and a sodium overload will very quickly cause an increase in circulating blood volume which could embarrass the heart following restoration of spontaneous contractions. There are commercial solutions of sodium bicarbonate available containing 500 mEq per ml, but in moments of stress it is quite impractical to monitor a proportion from such a large volume, and large containers should not be used for this reason.

Fibrillation may persist in spite of correction of the acidosis. If the fibrillatory waveform is a fine one it may be rendered more coarse by the action of adrenaline. Coarse fibrillation is more responsive to defibrillation than the fine variety so 10 ml of 1 in 10,000 adrenaline should be given intravenously. If fibrillation persists in the presence of a coarse waveform, an anti-dysrhythmic drug may be effective, eg. lignocaine 100 mg, bretylium tosylate 300 mg, phenytoin 100–200 mg, magnesium sulphate up to 10 ml of a 50% solution. Anti-dysrhythmic drugs may impair the contractility of the myocardium however so they must be used with caution.

Following successful defibrillation, it is usual to attempt to prevent a recurrence by continuing the administration of anti-dysrhythmic drugs. These must be given intravenously until the patient is able to take them satisfactorily by mouth, and may be continued for up to four weeks.

An effective cardiac output

The heart can nearly always be defibrillated even after prolonged periods of arrest of up to an hour provided that ventilation and cardiac compression are effective. Unfortunately, although patients may survive such a long period of resuscitation, there is no doubt that effective cardiac contraction following defibrillation is much more difficult to achieve when resuscitation has been prolonged. Failure to achieve palpable peripheral pulses from co-ordinated rhythm after 5–10 minutes is ominous. Calcium chloride

10 ml of 10% may stimulate the heart to produce palpable pulses without the support of cardiac massage but in the majority of cases, this response is transitory. Other stimulants can be tried as a desperate measure, e.g. isoprenaline, but any beneficial effect they may have is mostly overcome by adverse effects of an increase in heart rate and oxygen consumption. At this stage, for one reason or another, the myocardial fibres are unable to contract sufficiently to expel enough blood from the heart.

Asystole usually indicates massive heart damage,
> e.g. massive necrosis of the anterior wall and septum, involving both bundle branches. It is possible that a ventricular pacemaker will arise but it will be slow and unreliable. Artificial pacing is vital but the survival rate is very poor.

Asystole may follow an inferior infarction which interrupts both bundles but produces relatively little muscle damage. There is therefore complete heart block, but since the ventricles are in reasonable shape, any reliable pacemaker which emerges will maintain a spontaneous effective contraction. Pacing is not often necessary unless

1) the heart rate is unduly slow
2) there are brief recurrent episodes of asystole
3) the subsidiary pacemaker is in an unsatisfactory focus as shown by an unduly wide QRS complex, indicating that ventricular excitation is slow and uneven.

Occasionally, a subsidiary pacemaker fails to emerge spontaneously. The heart can often be stimulated to contract by sharp blows to the praecordium. This may lead to spontaneous effective contractions but if not, 10 ml of 10% calcium chloride or an infusion of isoprenaline may succeed. Isoprenaline 2.5 mg is diluted in 500 ml of 5% Dextrose and the infusion rate increased until a response is achieved, at which point it must be immediately reduced to avoid inducing fibrillation.

If all these fail, a pervenous pacing electrode will be inserted as rapidly as possible. If the heart can be 'paced' by blows to the chest and produces an effective output, and if distance and transport are a practical proposition, the patient can be transferred to the nearest available screening facilities for insertion of the pacemaker. If screening facilities are not available or continuous external cardiac massage makes screening impractical, a suitable wire electrode can be inserted at the bedside via the subclavian or internal jugular veins and its passage into the right ventricle monitored by the changes in an intracardiac ECG recorded from the tip of the electrode.

External cardiac massage

If cardiac massage is not performed correctly, it will be ineffective and will probably injure the patient.

Potential complications are:

1) fractured ribs
2) fractured sternum
3) contusion of the lungs and heart
4) rupture of the liver or spleen

In the majority of cases, such injuries result from pressure applied in the wrong place and in the wrong way.

Palpate the costal margin and identify the lower half of the sternum — in thin patients, this is not difficult, but in short, well covered patients, the lower half of the sternum is often much higher up than one would think.

The heel of one hand is placed over the lower third or half of the sternum, according to the size of the patient, and the heel of the other hand is placed on top of the first. Maximum even pressure is obtained if the hands are crossed at right angles to each other; in this position, the hands are in line with the forearms, although bent at the wrists, and it is easy to *keep the fingers straight.*

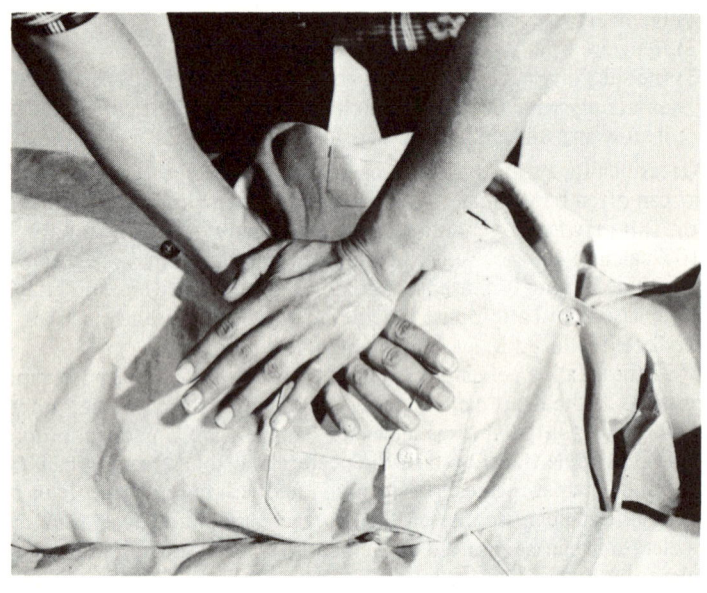

Fig. 17.5

The arms are kept straight, and pressure should be applied in a *vertical direction from the shoulders* to the hands.

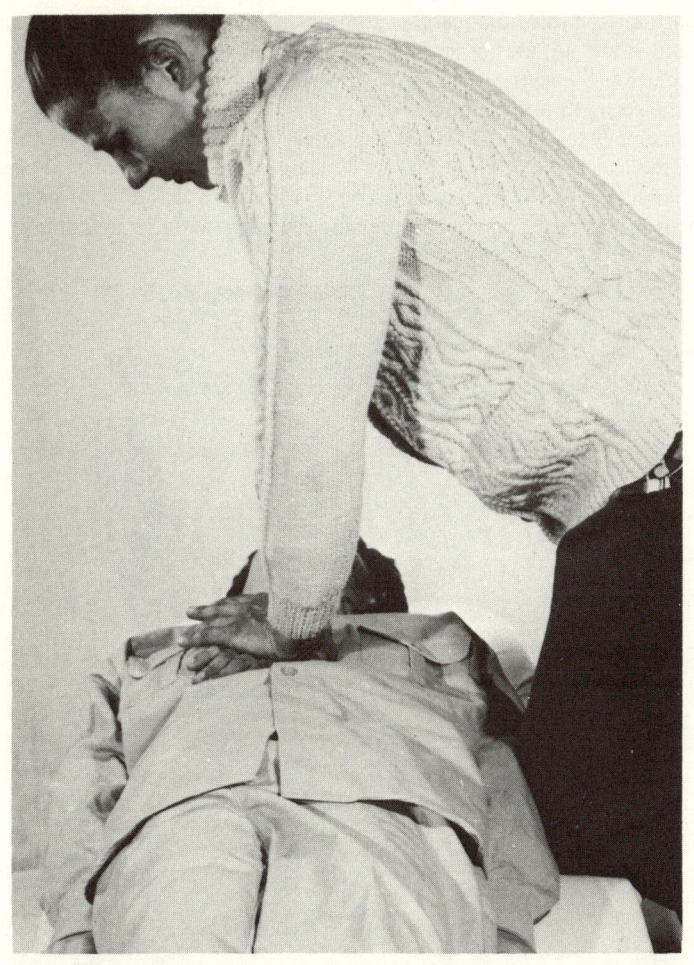

Fig. 17.6 External cardiac massage showing vertical line of force from shoulders to hands.

This means that you will have to kneel on the bed in order to bring your shoulders over the patient's chest. It is important, though, because it is much easier to compress the heart efficiently between the sternum and the vertebral column in this way. Few people are able to compress the heart effectively for more than a minute or two if they are *standing beside* a patient in a hospital bed. The mechanical disadvantage is such that most people soon begin to push laterally as well as down and the compression is less effective. Kneeling on the bed so that the shoulders are over the patient's chest means that cardiac compression can be continued efficiently for quite a few minutes by even the smallest nurse, because she is then able to use the *weight* of her body, through her shoulders and arms, rather than the strength of her muscles alone.

Remember to keep the fingers absolutely straight and do not let them touch the chest wall at any time. By concentrating on this, you will ensure that pressure is restricted to an area not greater than that of your palm — and this means that you are compressing the chest with the maximum

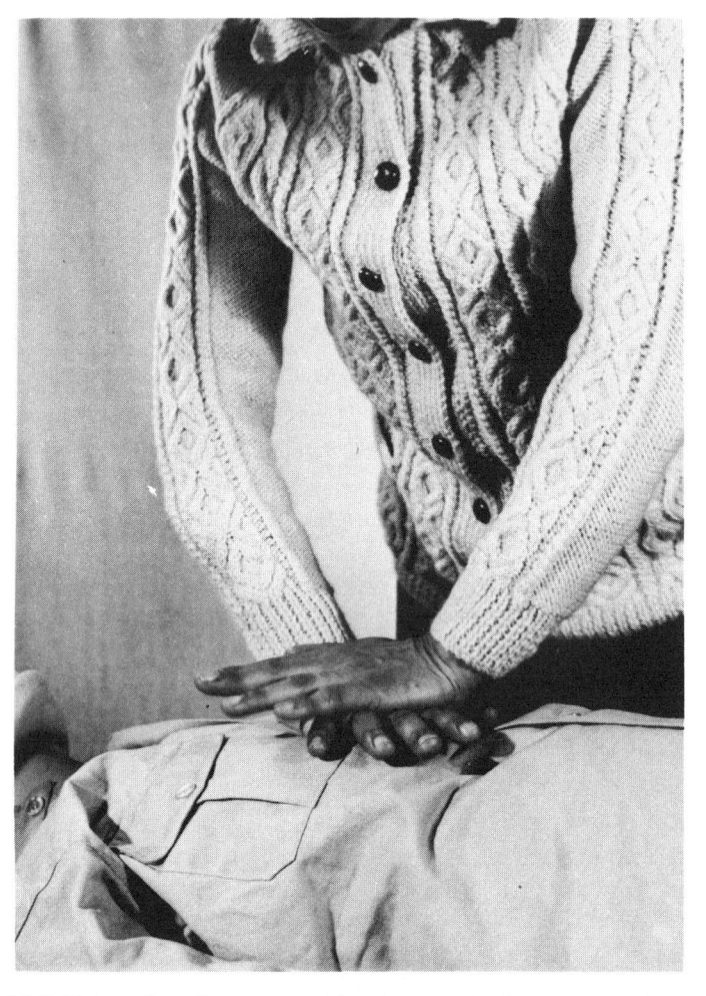

Fig. 17.7 External cardiac massage showing straight fingers, kept off chest.

amount of efficiency with the minimum amount of effort *and* are most unlikely to cause any damage to the patient.

Potential problems associated with ventilation of the lungs using a face mask and resuscitator bag are discussed in the chapter on acute respiratory failure.

Cerebral oedema

Any prolonged period of circulatory arrest causes cerebral oedema, which further reduces cerebral blood flow. Any patient who has had more than a brief period of cardiac arrest should be given 100 ml of 10% mannitol intravenously (or the equivalent) followed subsequently by 8 mg dexamethasone.

Subsequent management

Ideally, the patient in the general ward should be transferred to the coronary or intensive care unit following successful resuscitation, so that ECG monitoring, frequent assessment of the cardiovascular state and administration of anti-dysrhythmic drugs may be continued. If spontaneous ventilation is inadequate, the patient will require mechanical ventilation, if only for a few hours. Oxygen must be given in order to combat changes in the ventilation/perfusion ratio resulting from the effects of the circulatory arrest and also from possible lung contusion. If the patient has recovered consciousnes it is inhumane to withhold sedation and this should be given as required.

The prognosis for patients who have not recovered consciousness within 24 hours is poor.

Index

Acetylcholine, 79–80
Acid-base balance, 107, 111
Acidaemia, 183
Acidosis, 111
    metabolic, 112, 154, 177, 212
    respiratory, 111
Acids, 101, 107, 112
    strong, 108
ADH, 182
Administration, xii
Adrenaline, 68, 212
Airway obstruction, 38, 197–200, 201
Alarms, 139
Aldosterone, 181
Alkalaemia, 114
Alkalosis, 111
    metabolic, 113
    respiratory, 113
Alveolar oedema, 142
Ambu bag, 20, 22, 25, 209
Amino acids, 92–4
Aminophylline, 68, 143
Ammonia, 181
Ammonium ion, 108
Ampicillin, 68

Anaesthesia and anaesthetics, 28, 31, 76, 77, 88
Analgesia and analgesics, xi, 76, 78, 82, 84, 136
Anectine, 87
Anemometer, 7
Anions, 128
Ansolysen, 82
Anti-cholinesterase, 79, 86
Anti-convulsant, 84
Anti-emetics, 78
Anuria, 183
Arfonad, 89
Arterial blood gas measurement, 14, 103
Arterial blood pressure
    direct measurement, 44–5
    measurement of, 39–47
Arterial emboli, 145
Arterial oxygen saturation, 99
Arterial oxygen tension, 98, 100, 106
Arterio-venous fistula, 194
Aspiration pneumonitis, 71
Asthma, 68, 85
Asystole, 148, 151, 207, 211, 213
Atomic number, 115–116
Atomic weight, 116

Index

Atoms, 101, 115, 116
Atrial contractions, premature, 160
Atrial dysrhythmias, 160
Atrial fibrillation, 72, 163–5
Atrial flutter, 162
Atrial pressure
    left, 48, 49, 50, 137, 141
    right, 48, 49, 50, 51, 59, 137, 141
Atrial septal defect, 49
Atrial tachycardia, paroxysmal, 161
Atrio-ventricular block, 150
Atrio-ventricular bundle, 129
Atrio-ventricular node, 129, 150, 162, 163, 165
    abnormal conduction, 168
Atropine, 69, 78, 80, 151, 152, 159

Bacterial filter, 94
Base deficit, 106
Base excess, 106
Bases, 101, 107
Becton-Dickson Venous Pressure Manometer, 52
Benzyl penicillin, xi
Bicarbonate ions, 102–3, 105, 112
Bladder, care of, 24
Blood, 119
    carbon dioxide, 102
    carbon dioxide tension, 14, 105, 111, 202
    oxygen, 98
    sodium concentration, 119
Blood flow through kidney, 181
Blood gas measurement, 103
Blood gas tension, 103
Blood loss, CVP readings following, 59–61
Blood pressure, 136
    see also Arterial; Venous
Blood sampling, 137
Body fluids, 125
Body water, 184
Boiling point, 95
Bolus dose, xi

Bretylium tosylate, 150, 212
Brietal, 77
Bronchodilator, 74
Bronchoscopy, 200
Bronchospasm, 68, 75
Brook airway, 199, 203, 207, 210
Buffers, 109, 110
Bundle branch block, 175
Bundle of His, 129, 175
Bupivacaine, 69
Butyrophenones, 73

Calcium chloride, 70, 179, 207, 212
Calorie replacement in diet, 91
Calorie requirements in diet, 90
Cannula, 46, 47, 104, 194
    leaks, 47
    obstruction, 47
Carbenicillin, 70
Carbohydrate, 90, 91
Carbon dioxide
    excretion, 109–10
    in blood, 102
    partial pressure, 113
Carbon dioxide tension, 14, 105, 111, 202
Carbonic acid, 108, 109, 110, 112
Cardiac arrest, 135, 138, 153, 177
    conditions associated with, 208
    emergency procedure, 208
    outside specialised treatment areas, 203–17
    see also Heart
Cardiac glycosides, 72
Cardiac massage, 177, 200, 204, 207, 208, 210, 211, 213–17
    potential complications, 214
Cardiac muscle, 150
Cardiac output, effective, 212
Cardiac tamponade, 146
Cardiogenic shock, 144
Cardioversion, 72
Catheter
    bladder 24, 183, 185

Index

Catheter (*contd.*)
   Drum Cartridge, 54
   intravenous feeding, 94
   left atrial pressure, 137
   Swan-Ganz Balloon, 48
   tracheal suction, 20, 36, 37
   venous pressure, 48, 53
Catheter mount, 34, 36
Cations, 128
Cell, polarised, 128
Cell membrane
   polarity, 128
   potential difference, 128
Central venous pressure, 49, 50, 187
   following acute blood loss, 59–61
   high, 59
   low, 59
   measurement, 50
   taking a reading, 57
   within normal range, 59
Cephaloridine, 70
Cephalothin, 70
Cephorin, 70
Cerebral emboli, 145
Cerebral necrosis, 203
Cerebral oedema, 71, 217
Charts, xiii, 6
Chloramphenicol, 70
Chloromycetin, 70
Cholinesterase, 79
Cilial activity, 18, 19
Cleaning, 4
Clothing, 3
Compensatory pause, 172
Concentration, 65
Conduction block, 178
Conductivity, 129
Constrictive pericarditis, 49
Continuity of care, xiv
Coramine, 80
Coronary care unit, 135–47
Cortisol, 71
Coughing, 19, 20, 26, 38
Cuff inflation, 30

Curare, 89

DC shock, 151, 153, 154, 162, 163, 165, 167, 174, 177, 207, 210
Decadron, 71
Decimal system, 62
Defibrillation, 140, 153–5, 176, 205–6, 207, 210, 211, 212
Dehydration, 187
Density, 118
Depolarisation, 129, 130, 163
Dexamethasone, 71
Dextrose, 91, 191, 213
Dialysis, 188–94
Diamorphine, 136
Diastolic pressure, 40, 43
Diazepam, 71, 76, 136, 174
Diet, 187
   calorie replacement, 91
   calorie requirements, 90
   protein replacement, 92
   vitamin requirements, 94
Diffusion, 122, 188
Digitalis, 151, 188
Digoxin, xi, 72, 143, 162, 165
Di-hydrogen phosphate ion, 108
Dilantin, 84
Dissociation, 108–9
Distal convoluted tubule, 181
Diuretic, 74
Domestic duties, 4
Dopram, 73
Doxapram, 73
Droleptan, 73
Droperiodol, 73
Drug administration, x, 137
Drugs, 62–89
   anti-arrhythmic, 150
   anti-dysrhythmic, 138, 166, 167, 211, 212
   concentration, 65
   doses, 62
   list of, 67
   solutions, 65

Index

Drum Cartridge Catheter, 54
Duration of stay, xii-xiv
Dysrhythmias, 135, 136, 138, 141, 156–79
   following myocardial infarction, 148–55
   junctional, 165
   through abnormal AV node conduction, 168

ECG, 127–34, 136, 138
   analysis, 133, 157
   asystole, 213
   atrial flutter, 163
   bundle branch block, 175
   cardiac arrest, 210
   cerebrovascular accident, 145
   heart block
      first degree, 169
      second degree, 169
      third degree, 170
   junctional tachycardia, 167
   leads, 132
   monitoring, 45, 49–50, 135–140, 152, 154
   normal, 130
   physiological basis, 128
   premature junctional beats, 166
   premature ventricular beats, 173
   ventricular fibrillation, 154, 176
Ectopic pacemaker, 133
Electrode, 131, 152
Electrode jelly, 155, 176, 210–11, 214
Electrolytes, 101, 117, 120, 124, 184, 192
Electromanometer, 45–7
Electrons, 101, 115
Electroversion, 151
Elements, 101, 115, 116
Emergency boxes, 203–5
Endotracheal intubation, 5
Endotracheal tubes, 28–38
   nasal, 30
   oral, 28
   plastic oral, 28
   removal, 37
Epanutin, 84, 150
Ephedrine, 73–4
Epilepsy, 84
Equivalent weight, 120, 121
Eraldin, 85
Ethanol, 91, 92
Ethyl alcohol, 91
Extracellular fluid, 125
   osmolarity, 126
Extrasystole, 160
Eyes, care of, 24

Fat, 90–2
Fentanyl, 74
Fentazin, 83
Floxapen, 74
Flucloxacillin, 74
Fluid balance, 6
Fluid intake, 187
Fortral, 82
Fructose, 91
Frusemide, 74, 135, 143

Gases, 95, 117
   in solution, 96
   mixtures of, 96
Gastrointestinal tract, 24
Gentamycin, 74
Glomerular capsule, 180
Glomerular filtrate, 182
Glomerular filtration rate, 181
Glomerulus, 180
Glucagon, 75
Glucose, 91
Gram molecular weight, 118, 124
Gram molecule, 118

Haemodialysis, 193
   arterio-venous, 194
   veno-venous method, 193

Index

Haemoglobin, 98, 110
   saturation, 106
Haemophilus influenzae infections, 71
Hallucinations, 76
Heparinised saline, 45
Heart block
   first degree, 168, 169
   second degree, 168, 169
   third degree (or complete), 168, 170–2, 213
Heart damage, 213
Heart failure, 135, 142
   see also Cardiac
Heart muscle, 129
Heart rate, 133, 136, 157
Heparin, xi, 137
Heroin, 136
Hiccup, 24, 78
Hormones, 71, 75
Humidifier, 18, 27
Hydrochloric acid, 108
Hydrocortisone, 71
Hydrogen ion concentration, 104, 107, 110, 114
Hydrogen ions, 108–10, 112
Hypertonic solution, 190–2
Hypnotics, 81
Hypovolaemia, 60

Inderal, 85–6
Indomethcin, 146
Infection, 94
   of stoma, 35
   prevention of, x, 20
Inferior vena cava, 53, 193
Intermittent Positive Pressure Ventilation (IPPV), 5
Internal jugular vein, 54
Interstitial fluid, 126
Interstitial oedema, 142
Interventricular conduction defect, 134, 158
Intracellular fluid, 125

Intramedicut cannula-catheter system, 54
Intraval, 88
Intravenous feeding, 90–4
   basic requirements, 90
   complications, 94
   contra-indication, 94
Intravenous infusion, xi, 136
Ion exchange resins, 188
Ions, 101, 116, 117, 125, 128, 188, 191
Ischaemia, 168
Isoprenaline, xi, 75, 152, 179, 207, 213
Isotopes, 101

'Jack knife' position, 23
Junctional beats, premature, 165
Junctional rhythm, 167–8
Junctional tachycardia, 166
Junctional tissues, 165, 167

Keflin, 70
Ketaject, 76
Ketalar, 76
Ketamine, 76
Kidney, 180–95
   blood flow through, 181

Lanoxin, 72
Laryngoscopy, 200
Laryngotomy, 200
Lasix, 74
Left atrial pressure, 48, 49, 50, 137, 141
Left ventricular failure, 50, 68, 140, 142, 143
Lethidrone, 79
Levelling devices, 52
Levophed, 81
Liaison with other departments, xii
Lignocaine, xi, 72, 76, 150, 173, 212
Liquids, 95, 117
Lungs, 109
   compliance of, 7

Magnesium sulphate, 151
Mannitol, 76, 187
Marcaine, 69
Maxolon, 78
Miell, R., 1
Median cephalic vein, 54
Medical management, 4
Memory loops, 139
'Memory scope', 138
Mendelson's syndrome, 71
Mestinon, 86
Methadone, 77
Methedrine, 77
Methehexitone, 77
Methylamphetamine, 77
Metoclopramide, 78
Millimolar solution, 119
Minute volume, 7
Mogadon, 81
Molar solution, 119, 124
Molarity, 119, 120
Mole, 119
Molecular weight, 118, 119
Molecules, 95, 101, 116, 124, 125, 188
   number of, 119
   monitors, monitoring, 45, 49–50, 135–140, 152, 154
Morphine, 78–9, 136, 143, 162
Mulvein, J. T., 90
Muscle relaxant, 89
Myasthenia Gravis, 74, 80
Myocardial depression, 75
Myocardial disease, 49, 61
Myocardial infarction, 50, 75, 82, 135, 137, 140, 146
   convalescence, 146–7
   dysrhythmias following, 148–55
   major complications, 141

Nalorphine, 79, 84
Nasogastric feeds, 24
Neostigmine, 79, 89
Nephron, 180

Neuroleptanalgesia, 73
Neutrons, 101, 115
Next-of-kin, 3
Nikethamide, 80
Nitrazepam, 81
Nitrogen, 96
'No-touch' technique, xi
Noradrenaline, 81
Normal Saline, 120
Normal solution, 120
Nosworthy connections, 34
Nucleus, 115, 116

Oliguria, 183
   management, 186
Operidine, 84
Oradexon, 71
Oscilloscope, 127, 205–6
Oscillotonometer, 42
Osmitrol, 76
Osmolality, 186, 187
Osmolarity, 125, 185, 187, 191
   extracellular fluid, 126
Osmosis, 123
Osmotic diuresis, 77, 182
Osmotic effects, 124–5
Osmotic pressure, 123–4
Ouabain, 87
Oxygen
   administration, 136, 143, 167, 210, 217
   in air, 96
   in blood, 98
   mechanical ventilation, 22
   partial pressure, 97
Oxygen dissociation curve, 98
Oxygen release into tissues, 100
Oxygen saturation, arterial, 99, 138
Oxygen tension, 18, 27
   arterial, 98, 100, 106
Oxygen therapy, 138
Oxytetracycline, 88

Index

Pacemaker, 133, 149, 152, 160, 178, 213
Pain, 136, 146
Pancuronium, 81
Paroxysmal nocturnal dyspnoea, 142
Paroxysmal tachycardia, 160
Partial pressure, 96–7
Pathological specimens, xii
Patient
    attitude to, ix–x, 2
    conversing with, x
    psychological care, 2
    state of, ix
Pavulon, 81
Penbritin, 68
Penicillin, 68, 70, 74, 82
Pentazocine, 82
Pentolinium, 82
Pentothal, 88
Perfusion, 17, 60, 61, 99, 144, 145
Pericarditis, 146
Peritoneal dialysis, 189
    advantages, 192
    asepsis, 190
    complications, 192
    dialysate, 190
    duration, 192
Peritonitis, 190
Perphenazine, 83
Pethidine, 83, 136
pH value, 104, 105
Phenobarbitone, 84
Phenoperidine, 84
Phentolamine, 81, 84
Phenytoin, 84, 150
Physeptone, 77
Physiotherapy, xii, xiii, 20, 25
Plasma, 180–1
Plasma proteins, 125, 126
Polarisation, 128
Polarity, cell membrane, 128
Positive End Expiratory Pressure (PEEP), 5, 17
Post-operative care, xii–xiv

Potassium, 188
Potassium chloride, xi
Practolol, 85, 150
Pregnancy, toxaemia of, 72
Procaineamide, 85, 150
Propranalol, 75, 85–6
Prostigmine, 79
Protein, 90
    replacement in diet, 92
Proteus, 74
Protons, 101, 115, 116
Proximal convoluted tubule, 181
Pseudomonas, 74
Psychological care, 2
Pulmonary emboli, 144
Pulmonary oedema, 143
Pyopen, 70
Pyridostigmine, 86

Recovery area, xiii
Relatives, 3
Renal blood flow, 181
Renal damage, 187
Renal failure, 183, 191, 192
Repolarisation, 129, 130, 151
Respiratory failure, 196–202
Respirometer, 7
Resuscitation, 207
Resuscitator bag and face mask, 200–2, 217
Right atrial pressure, 48–51, 59, 137, 141
Right ventricular failure, 140
Rogitine, 84

Salbutamol, 86
Saline, 91
    normal, 120
Saline barrier, 44
Saline manometer, 50
Saliva, 23
Salt intake, 185
Saturation, 98
Scales, 52

Scribner shunt, 194
Secretions, 18
Sedation, 29, 84, 136
Semi-permeable membrane, 188, 193
Sino-atrial arrest, 159
Sino-atrial block, 159
Sinu-atrial node, 129, 158
Sinus bradycardia, 159
Sinus dysrhythmias, 158–60
Sinus rhythm, 133, 158
Sinus tachycardia, 159
Sister, 2
Sodium
   in blood, 119
   in extracellular fluid, 126
Sodium bicarbonate, 86, 177, 210, 212
Sodium ions, 185, 186, 192
Sodium nitroprusside, 87
Solids, 95, 117
Solutes, 182
Solutions, 65
   millimolar, 119
   molar, 119
   normal, 120
Solvent drag, 192
Sorbitol, 91
Sphygmomanometer, mercury, 39
Spirometers, 7
Sputum, 18, 19
Staff nurse, 2
Staffing, 1
Status epilepticus, 72
Sterile precautions, x
Sternal angle, 51
Sternal notch, 51
Steroid hormone, 71
Stoma, 26
   care of, 36
   infection of, 35
Streptomycin, 87
Strophanthin G, 87
Student nurses, 1
Subclavian vein, 55

Sublimaze, 74
Succinylcholine, 87
Suction, 29–30
   tracheal, 19–20, 35
Superior vena cava, 54
Suxamethonium, 87
Swan-Ganz Balloon Catheter, 48
Systolic pressure, 40–4

T piece for use during spontaneous respiration, 26
Tetracycline, 88, 188
Thermostat, 19
Thiopentone, 88
Thromboembolism, 144
Thrombophlebitis, 91, 94
Tidal volume, 7, 14, 15
Tissue perfusion and drugs, 137
Tracheal suction, 19–20, 35
Tracheostome, care of, 35
Tracheostomy, 5
   complications of, 38
Tracheostomy tubes, 31–4
   removal, 37
Tracheotome, 200
Tracheotomy, 200
Tranquillizers, 71, 84
Transducer, 45–6
Trimetaphan, 89
Tubarine, 89
Tubocurarine, 89
Typhoid fever, 71

Units, International system, 64
Uraemia, 183
Urea, 183, 187
Urine
   retention, 184
   specific gravity, 187
   specimens, 186

Valium, 71
Vapour, 95–6, 117
Vasoconstriction, 68, 78, 81
Vasodilatation, 68, 75, 84, 88

Index

Vasopressor, 78
Venous admixture, 99
    sources, 100
Venous pressure
    measurement of, 48–61
        scales and levelling devices, 52
Venous pressure manometer, 56
Ventilation, 99
    artificial 207–211, 217
    expired air, 198
    inadequate, 25, 29
    manual, 202
    mechanical, 5–27
    mouth-to-mouth, 199, 203
    mouth-to-nose, 198, 203
    short-term, 28
    spontaneous, 24, 25, 27
Ventilation/perfusion ratio, 99, 100, 217
Ventilation volume, measurement of, 6–14
Ventilator, 5–27
    controls, 5
    general nursing care, 22–4
    humidification, 28, 27
    negative phase, 17
    oxygen addition, 18, 22
    patient 'fighting', 16
    position of patient, 22
    positive end-expiratory pressure, 17
    settling patient on, 14–17
    suction, 19
    trigger sensitivity, 15–16

Ventolin, 86
Ventricular aneurism and rupture, 145
Ventricular asystole, 178–9
Ventricular beats, premature, 172
Ventricular dysrhythmias, 76, 85, 172
Ventricular failure
    left, 50, 68, 140, 141, 142, 143
    right, 140
Ventricular fibrillation, 138, 140, 148, 151, 153, 176, 207, 212
Ventricular rhythm, 133
Ventricular tachycardia, 149, 151
    paroxysmal, 174
Visiting, 3
Vitamin requirements in diet, 94

Wandering pacemaker, 160
Water
    distribution, 126
    in body, 125
    intake, 185
Water traps, 19
Water vapour, 96
Weak acids, 109
Wedge pressure, 49
Wenckebach phenomenon, 170
Wright respirometer, 7

X-rays, xii, xiii
Xylocaine, 76